To Die, or Not to Die

Praises for *To Die, or Not to Die*

"This book is full of helpful, practical information leading to patients gaining control in all aspects of their own healthcare. Creatively written with well-organized content and humor throughout. Very enlightening read!"

—**Jennifer Harrison**, RN

"This is a very informative book for women who want or need to learn the proper way to deal with modern medical situations when suddenly finding themselves on their own. I'm going to keep my copy on hand at all times."

—**Barbara J Lueking**

"A common sense approach to understanding and navigating the challenges of obtaining effective medical care. Tricks to Getting Better Medical Care is easy to understand and provides the reader with practical solutions in dealing with the many facets of the medical community."

—**Michael Harrison**, MBS, LPC

"This book is a must read. It provides patients with a complete guidance and follow through on their personal understanding of their health as well as dealing with day to day contact with health professionals. Dr. Cook's approach is magnificent, empowering people to understand their health and medical needs, taking them out of the void of following doctors' orders only and creating awareness of the backstage of doctors' lives and the medical system."

—**Ana Lioi**, CEO Mentor/Coach

To Die, or Not to Die

Ten Tricks to Getting BETTER Medical Care

JUDY COOK, MD

NEW YORK

BTo Die, or Not to Die
Ten Tricks to Getting BETTER Medical Care

Published in New York, New York, by Morgan James Publishing. Morgan James and The Entrepreneurial Publisher are trademarks of Morgan James, LLC. www.MorganJamesPublishing.com

The Morgan James Speakers Group can bring authors to your live event. For more information or to book an event visit The Morgan James Speakers Group at www.TheMorganJamesSpeakersGroup.com.

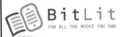

BitLit
FOR ALL THE BOOKS YOU OWN

FREE eBook edition for your existing eReader with purchase

_____
PRINT NAME ABOVE

For more information, instructions, restrictions, and to register your copy, go to www.bitlit.ca/readers/register or use your QR Reader to scan the barcode:

ISBN 978-1-61448-879-8 paperback
ISBN 978-1-61448-882-8 hard cover
ISBN 978-1-61448-880-4 eBook
Library of Congress Control Number:
2013947436

Cover Design by:
Rachel Lopez
www.r2cdesign.com

Interior Design by:
Bonnie Bushman
bonnie@caboodlegraphics.com

In an effort to support local communities, raise awareness and funds, Morgan James Publishing donates a percentage of all book sales for the life of each book to Habitat for Humanity Peninsula and Greater Williamsburg.

Get involved today, visit
www.MorganJamesBuilds.com

Habitat for Humanity
Peninsula and
Greater Williamsburg
Building Partner

To all the family, friends, colleagues, and patients
who have taught me so much in my life,
including
the importance of speaking out in their behalf.

Table of Contents

Foreword

Dear Reader:

I first met Dr. Judy Cook when she was a medical student where she was the brightest student in her class. Since she graduated from medical school, I have worked with her as a Physician, Pathologist and Psychiatrist. Dr. Cook never ceases to amaze me with her curiosity and is continuously searching for new challenges.

Her intuitive development of this patient guide book is a must read for patients, physicians and health care workers. The book shows common sense and is readily understood and fills a void in the market for an educational handbook to guide the patient to receive better, more cost effective treatment and involve the patient with his ultimate care.

Dr. Cook's book is unique, well written and concise and deserves a place in everybody's library. Physicians should donate "Ten Tricks" to their problem patients to create a better doctor-patient relationship!

Alain Marengo-Rowe, MD, FRCP, DCP, MRCP, MRCS, FACP

Preface

If you are not an educated, informed consumer of medical care and an active part of your own treatment team, you are at great risk for problems that may not only cost you money, but worsen your illness or even cost you your life!

A 2013 publication from the National Academy of Sciences shows that among the seventeen highly industrialized nations of the world, the US is among the richest and our health care is the costliest. Yet unfortunately, our results are usually among the worst.

Our lives are shortened more than that of other countries in areas of maternal conditions, communicable diseases, nutritional conditions, intentional injuries, unintentional injuries, drug-related causes, perinatal conditions, cardiovascular disease, and non-communicable diseases. Not only is the relative death rate higher, but the overall quality of life related to illness ranks lower than most of the other seventeen countries.

The approach of simply laying back and letting the health care team do what it wishes no longer works. Doctors have gradually moved away from being so available and authoritarian, so patients must move more into the role of being an active, informed participant in the decision making.

You are the person in your body. You have the best knowledge of your history of problems. You are the person who should be the most invested in knowing what is going on with your own medical diagnosis and treatment. The days of turning it all over to the doctors and letting them fix you are history, whether we like it or not.

The things I will recommend are not hard and fast rules. They are helpful guidelines. There will always be situations where things cannot, or should not, be applied (such as when you are alone and unconscious) or need to be modified (such as a parent who is responsible for a child's history, or a designated family member who is responsible for elder care or some other issue causing some degree of incompetency). However, this book involves issues and problems that occur every single day in doctors' offices, hospitals, and other medical facilities repeatedly. This book will give you specific guidelines to improve the process and the outcome for you or a loved one.

Many books and articles—ranging from the oldest to the latest— spell out *problems* with our medical care system. The book *Your Money or Your Life: Rx for the Medical Market Place,* written in 1971, reveals that the current health statistics cited earlier differ little from 42 years ago. Considerable information has also been written about all the changes that are happening in terms of new medicines and new technologies.

Little has been written about ways to help patients and families navigate the system more effectively and efficiently.

This book intends to help you understand some of the problems as viewed from both sides, and to teach you some better ways to cope with the system as it currently exists. This book is not intended to be a scholarly treatise, nor is it meant to cover everything. My goal is to point out that there are a lot of really simple, basic actions that anyone can take to get better health and health care for themselves. My wish is that, with this and several other recent books, patients will become educated and push for the changes that clearly will *not* come from inside the system. I will also be adding information periodically through my website. (www.godrjudy.com)

In 1984, Dr. Stanley Wohl wrote *The Medical Industrial Complex,* where he clearly spelled out the moves by which hospital chains, labs, nursing homes, pharmaceuticals, doctor groups, insurance companies, and other components became the darlings of Wall Street. The development of the Medical Industrial Complex left us with a business complex that cares as much about our physical health as Bernie Madoff cared about his clients' fiscal health. In the current system, patients and doctors come out at the low end of the priority scale. This *must change* for anything to get better.

Despite those economically driven changes, there are still many doctors who care and are devoted to caring for patients. Unfortunately, their lives have become more like that of a hamster spinning in a wheel. The doctors run faster and faster while they get fed less and less; this situation causes some to succumb to the problem in one way or another. Some join provider groups; some keep trying to run faster; others opt out of the system and go to cash only; some jump completely off the medical practice hamster wheel. Some of us are trying to find ways to improve the system. In my view, it is you—the consumer—who has to become the primary force to change things.

Although this is a country with a free market economy, where price should be driven by quality, consumer demand, and similar issues, no such market exists in medicine other than possibly in pharmacies and in plastic surgery. You do not *really* get to compare hospital prices, equipment prices, drug prices, doctor prices, or insurance prices the way you might compare the prices of cars, car repairs, groceries, clothing, or much of anything else. Furthermore, you are taught to depend on the system *to save your life* and not to question, just to pay. This allows the purveyors of medical care to continue to increase their charges while they continue to deliver less and less.

It is my hope to inflame a rebellion. I want you to learn to take better care of yourself, to learn the deceptive tricks and traps in the system, to recognize what you must do to protect your life, to decrease the demand on the system, and to force that free market economy to drive prices down.

Some ideas I discuss will seem obvious, or idiotic, or off the wall, but I can assure you, they stem from the kinds of issues doctors deal with in their offices and in hospitals on a regular basis. Unfortunately, I have never been good at creating fiction, so even though some of it may *seem* fictitious, welcome to a world that may sometimes seem stranger than fiction.

Introduction

Changing Times

The medical world is changing quickly. Good communication between doctor and patient is becoming even more important today than it has been in the past. The information you supply as the patient is critical to getting both optimum health care and the most help with the least amount of stress, effort, and frustration for both you and your doctor. The goal of this book is to give you some guidelines that will help in this process—and will also help (if enough people apply these principles) to decrease those horrible waits in the doctor's office that are brought on by not only the unexpected emergencies, but also the extra time needed to deal with some patients to clarify the needs and problems they present. Having yourself, your medical history, your current needs, and your current medications and other treatments more organized when you go in can help you and everyone else.

These guidelines will become increasingly important now that we have moved into a world where you may be "televiewing" with a physician at a distance and even having some examinations done via the medium of TV and computer with the aid of a nurse or other technical aide, rather than in the physical presence of the doctor. Sometimes the world of Star Trek seems to be drawing closer while contact with physicians is becoming more and more remote.

In the forty-plus years I have been in the medical field, the world of medicine has changed dramatically—some changes for better, some for much worse. There is no doubt that we have technologies, procedures, and medications that were totally undreamed of when I started school, or even a few years ago. A local 200-bed hospital recently acquired a robotic surgery device—the kind of (expensive) device that hopefully leads to smaller incisions, better treatment of specific lesions, and a shorter healing time, although current studies of results are giving less-than-glowing reviews. This kind of surgery may well move to outpatient surgical centers within a few years, as did many other techniques, such as laparoscopic surgery, that only started being used in the mid-1980s.

The diagnostic testing that can be accomplished now is incredible—whether it is automated chemistries, highly sophisticated and detailed radiology tools, or analyzing your genetic material. We have so many more medications to treat in so many more areas that—between the improved diagnostic techniques and the improved medications and treatments—we *should* be celebrating an incredible improvement in overall health and quality of life. It would also seem that with so many things available, doctors would have *more* time to spend with their patients and could continue to have time to care about their patients and to know them well. It would also seem reasonable for us to have some of the best medical care in the world.

However, we are a long way from delivering the best medical care in the world, ranking somewhere around *thirtieth* internationally in quality of health care, despite our relative wealth as a country and the extremely high cost of medical care and associated products. We rank below most of the other industrialized nations, regardless of whether that nation does—or does not—have socialized medicine. This problem has only continued to worsen in the years I have been in medicine. Despite health care reform, the prognosis for change remains fairly bleak, making it increasingly important for you to be an involved and proactive consumer.

The Medical Industrial Complex

Want to know why health care costs are high? To give you a thumbnail sketch, the Medical Industrial Complex has been developing for a long time, and when you add up all the associated costs and components, health care costs account for 17 percent of government spending. Once you add in all the privately funded medical care, it probably generates 20–30 percent of our gross national product. When all the associated components are combined, medicine as a field is probably one of the largest employers and contributors to the gross national product in the country.

It is easy to think of the medical system as only consisting of doctors and hospitals, but it is a vast and complex network. It includes the insurance companies, pharmaceutical companies, pharmacies, laboratories, X-ray and radiology facilities, equipment and supply manufacturers, nursing homes, rehabilitation facilities, and publishers of books and journals. Personnel also includes nurses, technicians, pharmacists, dieticians, chiropractors, physical therapists, occupational therapists, counselors, secretaries, office managers, dentists, opticians, and others. It also requires its own array of support in terms of advertising media, buildings, real estate, utilities, computers and IT personnel, food services, and delivery and transport personnel. While many of these items pull from other industries, they would not have nearly the business without the needs of the health care system.

Although the inclination is to blame doctors for that high cost of medical care, they are responsible for less than 2 percent of the total expenditures for medical care and probably considerably less than 2 percent of those "employed" in the medical system.

If one looks at a listing of the Forbes 400 richest people in America, there are only five doctors listed there. They include Dr. Bill Frist and Dr. Thomas Frist, who owned the Hospital Corporation of America hospital chain and held high national political office. Two others made their money with pharmaceuticals and one with medical equipment patents. The big moneymakers in medicine are the people involved in making decisions, laying out protocols, and running things like insurance companies, hospitals, pharmaceutical companies and equipment companies. In fact, they don't just make the most money. They make *most of* the money. They have also become quite talented at selling sickness rather than promoting wellness.

Why is any of this a problem? We have a system that employs many people and is a major component of our economic system— sounds like a great win. In theory, it could be a great win, but we only need to look at the cost, and where we rank in the quality of care compared to other developed countries in the world, and we begin to suspect there is a problem. The problem is that we have moved from a primarily patient care model, which was financially inefficient, to a complex business model that includes the insurance companies, hospitals, pharmaceutical companies, and equipment companies. This results in a model that has little concern about your physical or financial health. Not only is it all about the money—your money— but they play a shell game with the money where each handily blames the other for the need to keep raising their prices, and they all want to blame the doctors—plus or minus the lawyers and their lawsuits—for all the high costs. The balance has tipped from too little concern about the business of medical care to the other extreme.

Steven Brill's article "Bitter Pill: Why Medical Bills Are Killing Us," in the February 20, 2013, issue of *Time* magazine, does a wonderful expose of some of the problems with the prices, evasiveness and similar issues with most of the components, and laments that "insurance companies can't negotiate" with the other components.[1] What he apparently doesn't know is that there is no negotiating with insurance companies—they tell you what they are going to pay, and then they often renege on that and keep changing the rules for the other players. It is probably also a useful piece of historical trivia to know that Blue Cross Insurance (which only covered hospitals—the doctor coverage came many years later) was developed in 1929 at Baylor Hospital in Dallas, Texas (a church-related, nonprofit hospital). Might it be possible that insurance companies and hospitals have been in bed together ever since?

Also, over the past forty years or so, just as people as a whole are becoming less involved with each other directly because of the changing structure of society and a mobile work style and lifestyle, doctors are less likely to have a close, ongoing, working relationship with their patients. Even if they have the luxury of doing that, their time is still crimped, such that they have to see more people in less time than ever before.

This is brought about by many issues. These include but are not limited to the following:

- Insurance companies require more extra work, such as getting authorizations to perform treatments, hospitalize, or even to prescribe certain meds, which can take a great deal of extra doctor time and require the hiring of more staff. It almost seems as if the insurance company's goal is to save money

---

1   Steven Brill, "Bitter Pill: Why Medical Bills Are Killing Us," *Time*, February 20, 2013.

xx | To Die, or Not to Die

by *preventing* treatment rather than to improve health with preventive treatment.

- Not only do the insurance companies create a continuously increasing documentation load, but at the same time they are increasing your premiums, they are also decreasing payments to physicians when compared to the cost of living as a whole.
- Doctors have to see two to four times as many patients to make the same relative amount of money they used to make.
- There is a rapidly growing population with a declining percentage of physicians.
- Many people don't take care of themselves regarding prevention and management of chronic illnesses, which means they are in the doctor's office or the hospital more often.
- People all too often use a hospital emergency room to obtain care, meaning they get a new doctor each visit who does not know their individual health needs. This is not even close to optimum care.
- Patients (and often their families) have no concept of the time pressures doctors are under or that the doctor has additional patients. They often want to take enormous blocks of time to talk about things that frequently constitute chatty information best shared with friends.
- Patients sometimes don't comply with the treatment and then need to make repeated visits with the same problems, for which Medicare penalizes the doctors.
- Some patients make their own changes in meds either by not taking them or by adding something on their own, are not honest about it, and lead doctors to believe something is true when it isn't. Sometimes adding treatments could be harmful.
- Many over-the-counter meds can contribute to problems both on their own and by interaction with prescription medications.

- The extensive use of chemicals that can be abused, whether prescription or illegal, also complicates the scenario for a doctor and often leads to people being treated for totally the wrong ailments. This is particularly true as so many of these drugs are so easily obtained.
- Many mind-altering—and behavior-altering—drugs cannot be detected through the usual testing for drugs that can be abused. While the abuser may think he is pulling a fast one, it has also been known to cost him his life.

As if the above issues are not enough, many administrative changes have occurred in the use of computers, electronic health records, and electronic prescribing. While these can be good and useful things in the long run, for those doctors having to go through the transition, especially if they are not aggressively familiar with computers, it can be just one more component that sucks valuable time from an overloaded schedule and decreases the time and energy that can be spent with a patient.

Unsocialized Medicine

When I started practice thirty-two years ago as a psychiatrist, I could bill patients and insurance companies myself with a simple pegboard billing system. Insurance companies promptly paid me; my collection rate was about 95 percent; I charged and collected about $60 an hour for psychotherapy; and I scheduled my own patients. Currently, I have 1½ people as office staff and computers for each of them and myself. They handle billing and appointments, get treatments authorized, go back and rebill, and contact insurance companies repeatedly because they find ways to avoid or delay payment of claims.

Also, no matter what I charge an insurance company for a patient's visit, I will now get—thirty-two years later—about $105 for that same one-hour visit (but I will get $60 for a 15-*minute* visit). My current overall collection rate is about 50–55 percent because of mandatory insurance write-offs, and my overhead is *much* higher, since my staff ratio, space needs, rent, utilities, office supplies, and so on have considerably more than doubled (most things have increased about tenfold) in those same thirty-plus years. (Think 40 cents to $4 for a gallon of gasoline, 30 cents to $5 for a pack of cigarettes, and so on.) Since a psychiatric practice is much simpler to manage than that of probably any other specialty, and our overhead is lower than other specialties, this begins to give you an idea of what doctors in other specialties are dealing with and how it pushes the need to see more patients faster just to meet overhead. Clearly, the insurance companies—not the government—put the pressure on doctors to see people quickly and move through large numbers of patients if they are to make the kind of income most doctors hope to make after all the years of training and indebtedness acquired in going through training to be a doctor.

It may be of interest to you, as a carrier of private insurance, to know that your expensive insurance ties its payment rates close to the level of Medicare, so you pay a lot more, providers go through more hassles to be able to treat, and the doctor gets paid about the same—but the doctor has more hassle.

Socialized Medicine

Although I hear people complain about problems with socialized medicine, the socialized medicine we already formally have is Medicare, Medicaid, and the military/VA/Tri Care systems. It is much easier to get care for people under those systems than with the "unsocialized" system put in place by private insurance companies, who do far more to try to prevent treatment and payment for treatment than the "socialized" systems ever thought of.

However, the private insurance companies are edging their way into the "socialized" systems by being the "administrators" and wreaking havoc with them, too. Just as with private insurance, they are making it more difficult to justify treatment and get paid for it by both Medicaid and, to a lesser extent, Medicare. While I certainly agree there are problem issues out there that make surveillance and overview essential, this move is much more of an impediment to proper care than a resolution of those other problems. In his *Time* magazine article "Bitter Pill: Why Medical Bills Are Killing Us," author Steven Brill compares the cost for managing a claim for Medicare versus private insurance. Medicare was processing claims for $3 to $ 4 a claim, while it was $20 or more for the private insurer. Brill commented that the private insurers needed to bring down their costs, apparently oblivious to the fact that private insurance now administers Medicare and Medicaid and could lower that cost factor if they found it financially beneficial. It would be my thought that there was a bit of "skillful bookkeeping" going on here to falsely elevate their cost basis.

1

Be Your Own Advocate

For patients to get good care, they need to partner with their doctors and be actively involved in their own care in a constructive way that makes things flow more smoothly for everyone. In particular, patients must do some basic things: keep an organized record of their medications, list their current problems, and know their medical history. These simple things will take some of the time stress off the doctor and help the patient get the quality health care they need and—hopefully—also accomplish it at a reasonable price for the patient and a reasonable fee for the doctor. I urge you to learn the tricks in this book about ways to organize yourself and your own medical information so it will be easier for you to get the best treatment and also to learn useful information about more effective management of issues like prescription costs, how to look around for the best care for your problems, when to consider getting a second opinion, how to deal with your insurance company, and so on.

I cannot stress enough that *you* must be the one most vested in *your* health (and, sometimes, that of your loved ones). You are the only one whose health you have to worry about; your doctor has to worry about hundreds—or sometimes, thousands—of patients. You know your history up one side and down the other because yours is the only one you are focused on. However, even you will not recall every detail at any given time, so it is not realistic to expect your doctor to remember every detail of your history in the same depth you do—no matter how much she cares. In fact, patients all too often come for a visit and omit important complaints because they "just forgot" and bring up the issue on the way out of the room, or later on with the nurse—or not at all. It can be especially difficult for you to relate even all your *current* symptoms, much less past history, if you are really sick or in serious pain. The doctor's recordkeeping helps, if you are seeing the same doctor, but some things probably have changed since the history you gave the doctor a year or two ago. You might have remembered something important you hadn't remembered to share previously. Even though it may be in the chart, doctors rarely have time to sit down and review your *entire* chart, and you must be an active partner in the whole *history* and the whole *treatment* process.

It is important for you to have and to maintain a good record of your own history. Don't take it as an insult or a lack of caring on the part of the doctor, but rather be alert and point out to them things they may not remember. Medical care *needs* to be a teamwork situation, and teamwork does not mean you dump out a few facts and then the doctor takes care of everything else. You must be aware of how your disease is affecting you and how your meds or other treatments are affecting you, and report *your observations* to your doctor. It is up to the doctor to question you further, as needed, to decide how those threads may be tied together. While you *could* be having a reaction or side effect to a medication you have been on for ten years, for example, it is much more likely to be something else—like a more recent medication or something totally unrelated. The doctor needs to take your observations against his internal and external databases of facts and work to come to the best next step in your treatment. You, as a patient, need to understand that any given symptom you have could be an indicator of many different problems, not just a single one. Think, for example, of how many things you already know about that can cause a fever.

Ironically, it is amazing how little some patients seem to know or care about their own illness, medications, treatment of their illness, costs, etc. It is frustrating to ask a patient for a list of *all* of his medications, and he refers to a "little pink pill" or uses some equally unhelpful description. The patient not only doesn't know the name and strength of his medication, but he often doesn't know how he is supposed to take it, even though it is on the prescription bottle, and he doesn't know what it is for. Patients often know and care even less about their disease and what it means for them.

Thankfully, not all patients are that passive, but the percentage is high enough to be frustrating, especially when they are intelligent enough and educated enough to be able to do much better. It is also one more issue that takes up doctor time when meds have to be looked up, and research has to be done to determine information the patient should already know.

It is equally frustrating to deal with patients who come in, have heard a TV commercial touting a specific medication, and want to tell you what their diagnosis is, and what they should be taking —all based solely on that commercial. How much easier life would be if they paid that much attention to what the doctor tries to tell them. As a patient, you need to understand that those commercials are *designed to sell you a disease* you probably don't have which their medication will fix.

Also, some patients, to their credit, have been doing some research on their illness, so they understand it better. Using that information as a springboard for discussion can be productive. But when the patient comes in and acts as if the information he got off the Internet is the whole picture and that he knows more than the doctor does about the illness, it can be unproductive at best and destructive at worst.

Think about how you would feel if someone came in, armed with a small amount of information in your area of expertise, and wanted to tell you how to do your job. Advertising, and even valid medical articles, rarely present more than a small segment of relevant information. If medicine were as simple as TV commercials make it appear, doctors would not be needed at all. Few symptoms, alone or in a cluster, will tell you or the doctor that there is only one disease that could be causing your problems.

Educating either group of patients, be it the ones who need to be taught what they don't know or the ones who need motivation to learn *something,* can take a great deal of doctor time, which doctors often simply do not have. Sometimes the doctor or her staff can help, or she can refer you to useful and appropriate resources to study your issues further.

Many other issues in managing your health are *your* responsibility, not anyone else's. *You* are the one who has to keep your appointments, take your medications, make the lifestyle changes, and basically take those daily steps to care for your own health under the guidance of a physician. Doctors are with you only briefly. The rest of the providing of care is in *your* hands.

Part of the issue for all of us is to plan ahead so that family members will have each other's information in case one of you happens to be too ill, too young, or too old to do so for yourself. Obviously, parents provide this service for children until they are on their own; hopefully, you will keep a record to pass on to them.

The information in this book can help you do a better job of caring for yourself and/or your loved ones. Many issues I discuss will seem like no-brainers to some of you, but they are brought up here because they are issues that are seen in doctor's offices on a regular basis.

Your Important Issues to Manage

- Keep your appointments
- Know your medications
- Know your current complaints or problems
- Know your history
- Talk to your doctor openly and honestly
- Learn about your illness
- Learn about your meds and other treatments
- Follow your treatment plan; write down the instructions
- Monitor yourself for how well you do or don't respond to treatment
- Get adequate sleep and rest
- Get help with your stressors

2

Prevention, Prevention, Prevention!

The most important strides made in health care over the centuries have not been made in treatment; they have been made in prevention. That should be your main goal in terms of your health. Everything else that follows this chapter addresses what to do when prevention has not worked. I will list some of the many preventive things done by society and things you can do yourself, or with the aid of doctors and others, that should help you avoid the need to go to the doctor for more than well-person evaluations. Know, of course, that the whole of the Medical Industrial Complex (and probably many other big businesses in the world) would be much happier if you didn't do these things, because it will cut drastically into their income. The choice is yours to look out for them, or to look out for *you*.

The first thing you must do is to stop looking for a *magic* cure to anything that ails you. Instead, start looking for the magic in yourself, and the magic that can be accomplished by our society working to promote preventive maintenance. Some major steps to improve health have been the simple issues of clean water, sanitation and waste management, immunizations, removing trash, and removing sources of disease spread, such as mosquitos, fleas, and rodents.

Shortly after I started medical school, the doctors and the garbage collectors in New York City went on strike at the same time. In case you aren't sure, the garbage collectors were missed the most. Not only have we kept more people alive by those methods than with all our antibiotics, but you will read later how antibiotics are betraying us.

The human body is an incredible piece of equipment with marvelous abilities to heal itself under many difficult circumstances with a minimum of help. It can survive incredible insults, especially with some of the incredible tools we have now for treatment and healing—things that no one could have imagined surviving in the past. The presence of all those healing tools may have made people lax and lazy in terms of what they can and should do to protect this wonderful body so it has a minimal risk of disease to begin with.

Most people do not practice nearly the preventive care on themselves they practice on their cars!

If you have a new Mercedes or any other nice quality car, and if you are a reasonable, sensible person, you are going to do the maintenance on it that prevents serious breakdowns. You will take it in for fluid changes, make sure the radiator has water in it and the tires are full of air, and take it to the shop if it starts acting strangely or a button lights up. You will not throw corrosive chemicals on or in it, participate in demolition derbies just to see how tough it is, or try to jump the Grand Canyon with it. You will feed it the proper fuel, oil, water, and air for the tires and whatever else it needs to help it stay functioning and minimize the chances for things to go wrong. When things do go wrong in spite of all that, *that* is the time to take it for "treatment."

I am going to list, and briefly elaborate on, some of the choices you can and should do to maintain your body and your brain in good operating condition and minimize the need for medical care.

Water purification and trash control are items maintained by our government for a large part of our social system. Despite this, each of us needs to control our own personal trash, so we don't let it pile up and expose us to problems. Whether it is piles of trash attracting rodents and snakes, standing water that can breed mosquitoes, or items providing hazards in terms of falls, fires, and so on, we need to control our personal trash. There are water quality standards (which are much stricter in large cities than they are in small special utility districts) that tend to protect us from the more severe issues of dirt, bacteria, other life forms that could bring us harm, and some chemical contaminants. We face more problems now with chemicals that get into our water that are not checked for. These include things like pesticides that can leach into the aquifers, medications and illicit drugs that get into our water via our sewage system, and toxic chemicals dumped from manufacturing plants. These *can* be what gets cleaned out in the normal water purification process. However, I live in a rural community; all they do is add chlorine to the well water. The water not only is very alkaline, but has so much sodium in it that it kills my orchid plants and is a risk to people with heart disease. If you live in an area where there is any kind of concern like this, there are in-home water purification systems you can use to prevent problems in this area. These range from the water pitchers with filters you can get in the store all the way to reverse-osmosis systems from companies like Culligan that take almost anything you can imagine out of the water so it is nearly like distilled water.

Sanitation and waste management have been quite important in the prevention of the spread of disease in a wide array of different ways.

Proper sleep is a critical part of staying healthy. It helps your mind and body cope and heal. It is an extremely important part of treating patients with any physical or mental illness. Poor sleep can cause a wide array of problems all by itself, whether for the short term or the long term. It has been known to cause people to have hallucinations, anxiety, weight gain, depression, cardiovascular problems, poor work and school function, increased pain, delayed healing, and a wide array of other chronic wear-and-tear problems for both the body and the brain.

Take time to relax and enjoy yourself, your family, and your friends. We are human *beings*, not human *doings*. Any failure to take care of the human side of ourselves—the emotional side of ourselves—is a major cause of both physical and emotional *dis*-ease. Good mental and emotional health is a cornerstone of ongoing good physical health. Failure to take care of yourself emotionally often causes you to neglect yourself in many of the important preventive areas listed above. It also lowers the ability of your immune system and other parts of your body to be able to maintain a state of good health. (See section on mental health in chapter 10.)

Hand washing is an important way to avoid spreading many kinds of organisms. If you are dealing with your own health issues, such as wounds you are in contact with, if you are covering your mouth while coughing, or if you are around people who are clearly ill and contaminating surfaces around you, then washing your hands well with soap and water is a good procedure to follow and is more effective than other kinds of hand sanitizers. However, you do not need to be frantic about the fact that everything you touch has germs. Germs are a normal part of life, a major component of our bodies and everything else on the planet, and exposure to them is an important part of developing a healthy immune system that helps us fight off those few types of bacteria that are harmful.

Immunizations are important. There is no significant evidence that they, or the thimerosal that has been used as a preservative in vaccines, causes autism. (We will discuss autism later.) The evidence is indisputable that millions of lives have been saved by preventing those severe diseases (with the possible exception of influenza). Although I was fortunate enough not to live in the era of smallpox, polio was an issue when I was young and too many people died, were crippled, or wound up in iron lungs. Those things don't happen with polio now because of the ability to immunize people. The vast numbers of the lives that immunizations save are well worth the risks they represent in terms of fairly rare complications. Frankly, you will be hard pressed to find *anything* in life that doesn't have some risk of complication— even breathing.

When I was in medical school in San Antonio, Texas, we had an outbreak of diphtheria that sickened and killed many people. It occurred because a segment of the population did not understand the value of immunizations and had never been immunized for diphtheria. They also didn't understand that sharing water from a common drinking vessel at a community well could spread disease from a sick person to a healthy one. These were totally preventable cases of illness and death.

We currently have a grossly underpublicized recurrence of whooping cough in this country. It occurs because so many parents are refusing to immunize their children; immunity tends to diminish as we get older, especially into our fifties. In babies, whooping cough can be fatal. In older children and older adults, it presents the problem of a severe chronic cough for about six months, one that cannot be treated with medication and that may lead to things like hernias and broken ribs.

England is currently having epidemics of measles because about 20 percent of the population has not been immunized, and the country is now mandating immunizations. Measles can and does kill people. One doesn't need to see many events like this to appreciate how such a simple thing saves many lives from being needlessly lost.

Cover your mouth or nose when you cough or sneeze. Use a cloth or tissue whenever possible since it does more to prevent spraying droplets from you to others. This health and courtesy measure is important, especially if you are sick with something infectious rather than dealing with an allergy.

Cover wounds that are open or appear infected. This is an important measure that helps to prevent getting an infection or spreading one. One problem with the MRSA is that it is all too often spread by people with open, infected wounds that they don't cover, because they seem to have no sense of the risk to others.

Eat healthy and maintain a reasonable weight. This advice will help you minimize issues with many different problems, including high blood pressure, diabetes, orthopedic problems, etc. Getting healthier, more appropriate foods and other nutrients into your system will go a long way generally to improve both your physical health and your mental well-being.

Keep your body physically active. When you stay active, it helps you maintain a better weight, but it also helps your overall physical and mental health. Our bodies are not designed to be inactive and tend to deteriorate in a number of ways if we are inactive. Physical activity also stimulates your brain, helps your intellectual capacity, and improves your emotional wellness. This is a true "use it or lose it" situation.

Avoid falls. First, work to make yourself fall proof. Stay active enough to remain limber and maintain your ability to balance. If you have trouble standing on one leg without risk of fall, you need to work to rebuild this ability. Second, fall proof your environment. Taking this step does a lot to protect you from accidental injury, and it becomes especially important as people get older, are less nimble, have poorer vision, and are likelier to have serious injuries from falls. Night lights are an inexpensive aid to preventing falls at night.

Avoid the abuse of chemicals that can be harmful to your body or brain or fetus. A glass of wine can relax you, but a bottle of wine can set you up for DWI (or other problems)—and a case of beer or half gallon of hard liquor is a recipe for disaster. Many other drugs, alone or in combination, may not only cause you serious problems, but they kill too many people. These drugs include cocaine, methamphetamines, Xanax, and hydrocodone. Even the much-exalted marijuana slows your thinking, dulls your reflexes, and puts you at risk for things like car wrecks.

Also, it is imperative that you not shoot up drugs or share drug needles unless you want to catch a life-threatening disease.

Do not drive if you must use intoxicating chemicals. This includes any prescription medication that might impair your ability to function because it makes you drowsy, confused, or less attentive. Do not drive and put the lives of yourself and others at needless risk.

Practice safe sex. It is far easier to live with the inconvenience or discomfort of this than with a sexually acquired disease which may or may not be treatable, or to deal with a pregnancy you are not prepared for.

Talk with your doctor about keeping your prescription meds at the lowest number possible to do the job. To do this, the doctor needs to know *all* your medications. (See section on Dangers of Taking Too Many Medications in chapter 9.)

Think before you engage in high-risk activities that put you or others at risk for physical harm or illness and decide whether you *really* want to take those risks. If you just *have* to drive your car at high speeds, do it on a race track where you don't put the lives of so many other innocent drivers at risk as you would if you were to do the same thing on a freeway. If you just have to do wheelies on your motorcycle at 80 miles per hour, don't do it on the freeway where you will distract other drivers and put them at risk. It's bad enough to take stupid risks with your own life, but you don't have the right to do that to others.

Don't take antibiotics unless you truly need them. They can set you up for acquiring worse infections and other complications in the long run. (See section on antibiotics in chapter 9.)

Treat insect vectors and habitats. While treating insect vectors of diseases, like malaria and encephalitis, may seem like some remnant from the past, not only is malaria still a major problem in areas of Africa where mosquitos abound, but encephalitis was an issue in 2012 in Dallas, Texas, and probably other metropolitan areas. It became necessary to spray certain geographic areas to control mosquitos because of the emergence of an encephalitis outbreak that was causing illness and death.

Important Prevention Issues

- Clean water
- Sanitation and waste management
- Trash control
- Proper sleep
- Take time to relax and enjoy yourself and your life
- Hand washing
- Immunizations
- Cover your mouth when coughing or sneezing
- Cover wounds
- Eat in a healthy fashion
- Keep your body physically active
- Avoid falls
- Avoid abuse of harmful chemicals
- Do not use mind-altering chemicals and drive
- Minimize other overly risky behaviors

- Practice safe sex
- Talk to your doctor about keeping your number of meds at a minimum
- Minimize use of antibiotics
- Control insect populations

3

How to Find
Medical Care Providers

To find a medical care provider—whether you need a physician, hospital, clinic, nursing home, rehabilitation facility, home health care provider, or many other kinds of medical care—you have several routes to pursue. Unless you are paying out-of-pocket, the first step should be to call your insurance company. Ask for a list of doctors or other appropriate providers in their network. Your copay will be lower because the insurance company has some degree of contract with these providers. The insurance company *may* help you find providers for any number of services that you need, if it chooses to do so.

You can, of course, look in the Yellow Pages of the phone book under the listings of "Internists" and "Family Practice" for doctors and clinics and other medical services. You can in the same way look up any other medical service you are seeking. Locate the ones that seem more convenient. You should call and ask them for more information.

Here are a few examples of what to ask: (1) Do they treat the kind of problem you have? (2) Do they take your insurance (or what is the charge if you don't have insurance)? (3) How long does it take to get an appointment? It is important to verify that the medical practice treats what you need help with. While that may *seem* simple, even though I am listed as a psychiatrist, people frequently call my office, looking for family practice or some other specialty I don't practice.

Generally, you want to be cautious about a single doctor running a large Yellow Page advertisement that might be better suited to a large clinic. Any time a doctor's advertisement is flashy and makes wild promises, let your fingers walk in a different direction. There are also Internet Yellow Pages, but those are not inclusive listings since there are many different providers; most doctors are not going to pay to get listed in multiple directories which may or may not attract the clients they want.

A Google search may give you a thorough listing (it does in the town where I practice), or it may not. It will not provide much other than the basic listing information, but it is probably more reliable than some of the online Yellow Pages.

You can also go online to the website of your state's medical licensing board. Search for doctors of a particular specialty in a particular town. Not only will it list them for you with all their contact information, it will list where they went to medical school, where and when they did their residency, and whether there have been any problems that have been brought before the medical licensing board.

You may want to look for a clinic that has more than one doctor; this makes it easier to have someone there for you even on holidays, weekends, and when your regular doctor is out of town.

Having more than one doctor is especially important if you have an illness that may require frequent care, such as brittle diabetes. Some solo practice doctors now cover that problem by also having a physician's assistant or a nurse practitioner in the office with them who can handle many issues.

If you think you have a complex problem, a clinic that has doctors from several specialties may be a good idea, but it is certainly not necessary. These kinds of clinics are often associated with hospitals or medical centers. Obviously, if there is a hospital in town, there will be doctors and doctors' offices fairly closely allied with that hospital. They can often also give you a list of names and will often gladly give you their doctors' directory. Some hospitals have their own physician groups and may have a service that will help you get an appointment with someone in their group.

Friends, relatives, and neighbors that you like are often a good referral source and don't mind giving you their view of a doctor they do—or don't—like. That kind of checking around can sometimes provide helpful information. It can also be biased for a wide variety of reasons, so tread with caution.

You might also want to call the local medical society and ask for the names of doctors in a particular specialty. They probably won't give you recommendations, but the local medical society can give you a list of names. In some towns, there will be someone knowledgeable enough about the personalities of the various doctors to give you a little guidance as to who might be a better fit for you, but don't count on that happening—that is a rare event.

Similarly, you can contact a medical school if there is one in your area, and they may be able to give you the names of graduates or former faculty members who are practicing in town. Usually, you want to call the department for the specialty you are interested in, such as family practice, to get that information. Most medical schools also maintain their own clinics, sometimes only for indigent patients, but they often have one for private patients as well. These can be good clinics, especially if you have something more complicated or unusual. You may also need to be willing to be a teaching case to qualify. That means you might be treated by a resident or a fellow, or if a faculty person treats you, students, residents, and fellows may be present to observe and learn. There may also be an option to be just a private patient. I know that, as a senior resident, I had several private patients; that seemed to work well for them and for me. That model is often a good one and may be less expensive if you are a private-pay patient. Sometimes, you can just call the medical school's clinic and schedule an appointment while some require a referral from another doctor. That varies with the facility.

Resources for Finding Providers

- Check with your insurance company for covered providers
- Check Yellow Pages, both hard copy and online
- Do a Google search for local doctors
- Check with the State Licensing Board
- Check with local hospitals, clinics, and medical societies
- Check with an area medical school, both for referrals and as a place for treatment
- Check with friends, relatives, and neighbors

4

Selecting the Right Place for Your Medical Care

Emergency Rooms

The first thing I would like to stress here is that emergency rooms are *not* the place to go unless you have a health event that is truly an emergency. The emergency room is just that. It is for *emergencies*—like car wrecks, heart attacks, sudden changes in how your brain works (without having changed it with chemicals), broken bones, sudden bleeding that won't stop from places you shouldn't bleed from, allergic reactions, accidental poisonings, and things of that nature. If you have a true emergency—something that may well threaten your life or seriously and rapidly impair your health without rapid treatment—by all means go to the ER.

If you have more minor problems, do not clog the ER and cause delay of treatment for people who have real emergencies. The emergency room *should not* be used for your headache you've had for two weeks (unless it just drastically changed), or the cold you are a little uncomfortable with, or because you have just decided your blood pressure medicine isn't right, or your belly has been bothering you for a month (with no change in the discomfort level) and at 2 a.m. you decide to go to the emergency room, or for your sexually transmitted disease, or routine follow-up for your pregnancy, or any of the thousands of ailments for which you should go to either your own personal physician or a walk-in clinic. Don't take the risk that the doctors will be too overloaded with urgent, life-threatening medical issues to give your problem the treatment it needs and deserves.

Even when you have one of those true emergencies, you still need to follow up promptly after that ER visit with someone who will treat you on a regular basis. Making repeat visits to the ER for follow-up treatment of your problem does not provide you with proper care. Realize that the busier ERs are, the more likely it is that they can make mistakes in the diagnosis and treatment of even serious problems (doctors *are* human, after all). Continuing to go back there rather than getting promptly aligned with someone who can focus more intensely on you and your specific problem is not the best way to get treatment. Even people who work in the medical field and have a medical emergency don't always get proper treatment in the ER. The patient needs to be watchful about his own condition and whether it improves after that ER visit and where he needs to go next.

It is not my intent to be down on emergency rooms. I just want to make you aware that it is an acute, intense pressure cooker of diagnosis and treatment. The more issues there are going on in the ER, the more likely you are to have something overlooked or not be given the right diagnosis and/or treatment. If the next day you are feeling much better, or you are in the hospital getting the treatment you need by the other doctors, well and good. If you are not in the hospital and are continuing to have problems, you need to turn to a primary care physician.

I recently treated a patient who, in the last three years, had made ninety visits to our local ER. I have no doubt she had made similar numbers of visits to other area ERs, in addition to being an inpatient a *few* times for more serious issues. I suspect *most* of those visits could have been avoided. Her care would have been much better had she allied herself with a primary care physician. In addition, in these days of soaring medical costs, those ER visits probably cost the taxpayers $6,000 *each* (since she has Medicare), while an office visit would probably have cost a few hundred. Thus, she would have had better care that would have cost less money. Just as an aside, she is now having repeat admits to a psychiatric unit and appears to have found a new way to misuse the system.

Primary Care Providers

Ideally, you and everyone else should have someone whom you establish a relationship with as your primary care provider (PCP), or "regular doctor," and that is usually a general practitioner (GP) or an internal medicine practitioner (internist). This should be the doctor who gets to know you and your history as a whole person—they know what ails you from head to toe. They can then help you get to other specialists as needed and helpfully have that information funneled back to them so they have your full record. (I also try to have that full record as a psychiatrist.) They treat you as needed and coordinate other needed care so things happen as effectively and efficiently as possible. It is much easier if they have a baseline on who you are and what your problems have been for them to move forward quickly with whatever you need related to your current problem.

It is important that at least one of your doctors (and preferably all of them) has the full picture of what is going on with you and every medication (including OTC) you are taking. They should also know about every other doctor you are seeing and every significant illness you have—or have had.

It is important that your primary doctor be someone you like, trust, are comfortable with, and that feel you can be open about all your issues. If you find you aren't comfortable with or don't trust this doctor for whatever reason, you would do well to first discuss your problem with the doctor. It may just be a misunderstanding that can be resolved with a simple discussion. If that doesn't work, you should probably consider changing to a different doctor and find one that you are comfortable with, will be totally honest with, one you trust to give you the best, and one that will call in someone else when your problems exceed their expertise. (If you think *any* doctor knows *everything*, think again—there is just too much to know. If you think a group of symptoms can only represent one disease, you are mistaken. If it were that simple, we would never have needed doctors.) If you can't find *any* doctor that suits you, that is another whole set of problems you may have—and that means looking inside yourself.

Most of all, you need to have a doctor you can and will be totally honest with. If you tell your doctor only some of your issues and leave out facts because you are ashamed, embarrassed, doing something illegal like abusing drugs, or any other reason, you risk greater harm to yourself. You run the risk that you will get treatment you don't need or will not get the treatment you do need, either of which could cause you major medical problems. Many people worry that a doctor will look down on them if they know the whole truth, but a doctor's job is not to judge, it is to get you well. In addition, there is not likely to be much you are going to tell your doctor that they haven't heard before, probably from *many* other patients. When a patient does tell me something totally new, that tends to stimulate my curiosity and get me investigating how that may—or may not—be important, not cause me to judge them.

When you don't have a regular doctor, you need to find one. That can, however, take some time because so many doctors have busy schedules. Many have also quit taking those insurances that pay the least money for the greatest hassle both in providing patient care and in collecting fees.

I cannot overstress the importance of having a doctor you trust and are comfortable with. Studies conducted long ago showed that, generally, a patient does better when he has a doctor with a good bedside manner than he does with a physician who is extremely capable but difficult to relate to. This, of course, relates to the power the mind has in promoting and creating wellness independent of any other kind of treatment one might receive.

Walk-in Care Providers

While you are looking for a primary care provider, you may find yourself needing to use a walk-in clinic. This is a place you can go, usually without an appointment, where they just take care of the symptoms you have at the moment and are not involved in treating the whole person. Some of them are minimal clinics while some of them are equipped with lab and X-ray on site. Some clinics designate themselves as "urgent care clinics." Often they have longer hours than the walk-in clinics. Either type is adequate to go to when you have a fairly sudden onset problem that is *not* life threatening. They can also advise you when they think you have problems that require an ER or other more intensive care.

While they may be quite adequate for minor injuries and minor illnesses, they are less appropriate if you have other chronic problems that may not be getting managed like they should be. For example, if you go to one of these clinics because you have a urinary tract infection (UTI)—a seemingly simple issue—but you also have poorly managed diabetes, and your blood sugar is now really high, it becomes a not-so-simple issue to resolve. Both issues need to be treated, and a medical professional needs to determine a longer-term treatment plan. If you go in with a headache that has been really bad the last few days, and you are convinced it is a migraine but you have not been taking your blood pressure medicine like you should, and your blood pressure is really high, it becomes a more complicated case. By the way, high blood pressure is only one of the many serious things that can produce a severe headache.

While the doctors and nurses in these clinics are certainly trained in all these areas, they are also aware that these are illnesses that need to be treated more often and seen on a regular basis for more intensive treatment, not just a drop-in basis. You may be able to arrange with them to do that, but you are probably going to have to find a non-urgent care doctor to provide your ongoing treatment. Many walk-in clinics are equipped to do a wide range of basic lab studies and X-rays, but again they will just be looking at the more basic issues that need more immediate treatment.

There is a newer type of drop-in clinic starting to emerge, one that is basically staffed just by nurse practitioners and/or physician assistants with no onsite physician. They can handle a variety of routine issues, including chronic management of diseases like diabetes and hypertension, but they should refer you on if it gets complicated. In addition, many pharmacies are now expanding their services from a minor clinic for things like flu and pneumonia shots to a walk-in clinic with a nurse practitioner to help you manage your diabetes and blood pressure. They are going to be much more limited in terms of any ability to get laboratory tests or X-rays. They may also be under pressure to prescribe you meds you may not need at a "special deal" with the host pharmacy. They may be more convenient than seeing your regular doctor because of their hours and drop-in schedule, but if you have other more serious underlying medical issues, this may not be your best choice.

Be sure you let your PCP know when you have visited any of these clinics so the illness and treatment can be recorded in your medical history, and be sure to include it in your own medical history log.

Specialists

Specialists are doctors who have gone beyond general medical training to specialize in one area, and they don't try to treat or coordinate treatment for the whole body like a PCP does. They have much more intense information in their specialized area that they focus on. They are the people to go to once things are getting complex, and your PCP feels you need someone with training in a special area. There are many specialties, including cardiology (heart), hematology (blood), psychiatry (emotional), pulmonary (lungs), neurology (brain and nervous system), rheumatology (bone and joint illnesses, but not fractures), allergy, gastrointestinal (stomach and gut), surgery, and so on. In the specialty of surgery, there are many more subspecialties, including those who specialize in broken bones, backs, brains, hearts, eyes, ears, noses, throats, children, cosmetic repairs, and others. It is a long list. Your PCP is the coordinating physician, helping you get to the right specialist for your problem. This is an important part of good, effective, efficient medical care. It may also help steer you away from some procedures you don't really need, ones which might not benefit you but which some people would be happy to sell you anyway.

Interestingly, in Canada it is even more difficult to get in to specialists than in the US. The waiting list may be up to two years, even with the referral. Their socialized medicine has its problems in this area, but I do not know what the driving factors are there. Perhaps doctors don't specialize or don't get paid, or perhaps they come to the US where specialists make more money, or other issues. I also hear that basic medical care is better in Canada because patients are more conscientious about follow-up care.

In America we have a relative shortage of PCPs, such as in family practice, pediatrics, and internal medicine. This is probably because they are at the low end of the financial reimbursement ladder, despite being the foundation for good treatment. Specialists make three to four times as much money and often have an easier schedule. Paying primary care providers more and specialists less would probably help resolve this dilemma.

Whether good or bad, insurance companies have become more involved in putting limits on what treatments you can have (if they are going to pay for them), but they are not always as vested in your best medical interests as they are in their own best financial interests. However, even as a psychiatrist, I find it much easier to be an effective advocate with insurance companies or other doctors to get the kind of treatment a patient really needs when I know a patient well. It works much better than when I am dealing with someone I have just met and don't know that much about.

Sadly, the job is made more difficult for doctors and insurance by those people who seek treatment they don't really need. This fortunately fairly small group seems to make it a practice to abuse the system instead of using it for getting help just when it is needed. This faction contains the worried well, substance abusers, people trying to get disability benefits, people whose untreated emotional pain causes resistant physical pain, and other issues. It also includes people who could prevent a lot of treatment by proper lifestyle changes.

Ironically, one advantage of having the insurance companies manage care is that sometimes they are able to advise a doctor of the various treatments people have sought in other places and how frequently. This can help us immensely in knowing what treatments they have had, what medicines they are supposed to be on, and significant history, including getting meds from multiple physicians, which could be problematic. Hopefully, *that* will become a collaboration for treatment that will help to improve patient care over the years, but it is currently still a rare event, as is making good and useful data readily available by having electronic health records. This book will teach you some of the things *you* can do to make your collaboration with your doctor more productive in maintaining your good health.

It is important for you to make a point of being as aware as possible of everything that is going on with your health care. Know what treatments and tests have been done, the main points of the results, the medicines that have been tried (whether helpful, harmful, or just of no benefit), and other relevant history. Getting the doctor who is treating you up to speed with what has happened will help eliminate a lot of repeat testing and treatment and save more of your money and time.

Second Opinions

If you or your family are having some doubts about how you are being treated or about a recommended treatment, or you just want to be as sure as possible that there aren't other or better alternatives, don't hesitate to get a second opinion. Often your doctor will be willing to recommend someone, but if they aren't, then use the search options listed above. You can also look in another town, or check with a major facility or a medical school. Many people also want to look into alternative and naturopathic alternatives; these can be helpful. Certainly, doing some research yourself with the myriad of legitimate online resources will give you a sense of whether you need to spend the time and money it takes to be sure you are following the best option.

Treatment Options for the Underfunded

With so many people in our country uninsured and so many people in impoverished financial straits, many go to the ER for any kind of care they need because they know they cannot be refused there. However, that is changing. ERs will more and more freely deflect people who are not truly in need of emergency care to alternate facilities. In addition, they will bill you for using the ER whether you are indigent or not, and it will be much higher than going to a primary care doctor. (While they may never collect it, it will reflect on your credit history and get in your way if you are trying to move forward with your life financially, and you will probably have to deal with hostile collection agencies.)

Some clinics do work with lower income people, funded generally by a cooperative effort of local, state, and federal government to help those in need of care and unable to pay for it. Sadly, despite the attempts at medical care reform, it is getting more difficult for people who have Medicaid (and sometimes Medicare) to get help because of the low rates—which seem to be getting lower—that they pay to doctors and clinics. Some facilities have closed because they cannot meet overhead any more.

A great many people think that because they have insurance, the doctor or facility is paid at 100 percent. However, insurance companies decide what they will pay and what you are allowed to pay; the doctor or facility has to write off the rest of the charge, often 50–75 percent or more. This will probably necessitate more of these funded clinics, despite the press to have a larger percentage of the population insured.

Sometimes there are free neighborhood clinics set up in poorer neighborhoods, which usually are the result of donated time from doctors and nurses and donated resources from other types of providers. There are also places like United Way that will help you get medications, and places like Planned Parenthood that help women with all their health issues, not just issues related to reproduction. Drug companies have patient assistance programs to help you get your medication for free if you qualify based on your income.

However, it is also important that you, as a potential patient, keep in mind that if you can buy cigarettes and beer (or other substances that can be abused), can afford to take care of twenty stray animals, see yourself as a rescue service for wolves, or can keep bailing your children out of jail (no, I am not making any of this up), *you can make a better choice*. While I don't want to see anyone have to choose between food and medical care, I have little sympathy for people making choices like the ones I've just presented to you.

You can spend your money in more appropriate places, like buying healthy food. You can also pay for medical care that helps you stay healthy so you don't wind up causing more health problems for yourself. The benefit is that you feel better and also do not run up high medical bills that either give you problems or increase the tax load for everyone else inappropriately.

You also need to recognize that you will not get the first-class care that you would like when you cannot afford more than bargain basement prices, and when, in addition, you don't make taking good care of your health a priority. I don't go out and expect to buy a car I can't afford; instead, I will settle for a less expensive one that will still do the job, even if it isn't as fancy. I will then take good care of it, so it serves me well. I will strive to afford progressively better things. Similarly, people have to recognize that looking for the equivalent of Mercedes Benz medical care when they can't even afford a beat-up, used Ford truck level of care, is not realistic.

All patients from every economic level also have to start working with their doctors and clinics to make reasonable efforts to take care of themselves. They should take their medicine; watch their diet; avoid risky behaviors; get some reasonable physical activity; get adequate sleep; avoid drug, alcohol, and food abuse; keep their appointments; and other simple actions that will decrease the need for medical care and help them stay healthier at a lower cost.

Hospitals

Most people understand that hospitals are the place to turn to when your medical issues cannot be managed in the doctor's office. To get into a hospital, you must be admitted by a physician, preferably one who has been treating you regularly, and if not, via the ER physician if they decide admission is necessary. Thus, your choice in this area is determined by who you go to for care and what hospital they use, or by what emergency facility you go to. In the case of a 911 emergency, it will be the closest hospital available.

5

Preparing for Your Outpatient Visit

For Inpatient or Outpatient Visits

While this chapter addresses mostly outpatient care, the same issues are important for inpatient care as well. In the hospital there will be many additional issues to cope with because you will be more ill and will be in the midst of number of other patients who are seriously ill. There will be more exposure to infections and you will want to be more aware of good cleanliness practices. Staff may be quite overloaded at times and you may need to put out more effort to get their attention if you really need them urgently. The book *Design to Survive: 9 Ways an IKEA Approach Can Fix Health Care and Save Lives*, by Pat Mastors, may be worth your attention regarding inpatient care.

Whenever you are hospitalized, injured, feeling really bad, feeling confused or overwhelmed, or are considering some kind of procedure, take an advocate with you. This can be a family member, close friend, or caregiver. This person should also know what your problem is so if you forget something they can help give that history.

They can act as an aid to ask additional questions you might not think of and help remember the doctor's instructions. In the hospital they may need to be there to help you with personal care and attention or in summoning medical help. They may also be able to help you research your illness before you decide to have a procedure done.

Make a Simple List of Your Current Medical Complaints

When you call to make your appointment at any outpatient facility, it is a good idea to give the staff an idea of the extent of your problems so they know how urgent it is and whether to book you for fifteen minutes, thirty minutes, or even longer, and how soon you need to come in. If you are just scheduling a yearly check-up, you probably won't have any complaints. However, you do need to attend to the other items I will be addressing.

A good history goes a long way toward helping you get good care, and a poor history can cause you a lot of problems. Doctors are not veterinarians. They rely on your history to direct where they need to go for the physical exam and diagnostic studies. They don't have a magic scanner like the one on Star Trek. If they did, the current medical environment would make each scan cost a fortune. When you go into the doctor's office, you need to have a list of the pains and problems you are coming in about. When you are sick or in a great deal of pain, it can be difficult verbally to give a clear and simple list of what is bothering you and to remember all the items.

As your problems come up, and *before* you get to the doctor, write them down. Use the Current Complaint Form on my website (www.

godrjudy.com). Take it with you. It will also have room for you to write what the doctor tells you to do so you don't have to try to remember things when you don't feel good. Also, take a list of all your current meds, allergies and so on, and a copy of your abbreviated whole medical history. (Those forms are also on the website.)

Little is more frustrating to a doctor or the office staff—or more likely to impair a patient's care—than when the patient comes in for what should be a brief visit, perhaps fifteen minutes, and it takes thirty minutes of wading through a lengthy discussion of symptoms and history to even determine the patient's complaints and what she wants help with. The patients with the longest, vaguest list of complaints are also usually the ones who, once you have set up something, make a "by the way" comment as they are going out the door which finally gives a clue as to what the *real* problem is. That problem may be something totally different from, and more urgent than, what was being treated already, and requires a great deal more time. Yes, you can be rescheduled, but it may take time to do that and, meanwhile, you may not be getting the right treatment and might even get the wrong treatment. It also only takes one or two patients a day like that to throw off a doctor's schedule so that everyone else winds up waiting a long time.

When you go in to the doctor, have that list of things that are causing you distress so that you will be sure to discuss all the important issues so they can be checked out. Try to make some *brief* notes like what the symptom is; where in your body it is; how long has it been bothering you; what seems to make it worse or better; things that might have happened before the problem like an injury, another illness, a medication change, or an emotional or social stress. Be sure you also take a list of *all* your meds, including OTC ones, and it's a good idea to also know which ones you may need refilled or have doses adjusted. Check your history to see if there have been any changes since your last visit. Although keeping it brief might feel as if you are getting shortchanged, it is actually something that helps keep you and the doctor focused on the issues that are critical to getting you good care for your current problems. If you have chest pain or belly pain, or whatever might be causing your recent distress, stay focused on that issue. That is important in getting the care you need for the problem you have. The doctor will ask additional questions and do physical and lab to clarify what is going on, because things aren't always as simple as they seem.

For example, I have seen abdominal pain that turned out to be caused from diabetes, pneumonia, and other things that seem unconnected, just as I have seen emotional pain, such as apparent depression, come from a wide variety of medical illnesses, and physical pain or illness that is caused by emotional distress.

Also, please try to bathe before you come to the office. While it is understandable that you may feel sick and certainly don't want to dress up, cleaning your body is not only healthy for you, but a kindness to the office staff, the doctor, and the other patients in the waiting room. That may sound like a no-brainer, but I have had people come to my office smelling so bad I had to spray room deodorizer throughout my suite. They were not physically impaired; they just didn't attend to things like bathing and washing clothes regularly. I know there will be times when that is not a reasonable thing to ask, but most of the time people can do that.

Always Keep a List of Your Medications/Allergies with You

First and foremost, put together a record of your personal information that includes: name and address; emergency contacts; names and phone numbers of your doctors; a list of *all* of your medications, including all over the counter medications; list any allergies and any adverse medication reactions; and a list of your current illnesses.

Put this on a piece of paper you can carry with you, on your person, at all times.

Why?

Because, first, every doctor you have needs this information. Second, if you suddenly have a medical emergency and are unconscious, people will have access to urgent information to help you much more quickly and much more effectively. It is wise to also have copies with family or friends you trust. You can find a downloadable template for this form at www.godrjudy.com.

Know Your History (and Have It in a Written, Easy-to-Access Format)

I am a firm believer that everyone should keep at least a basic medical record and edit it any time something of any significance occurs. It is good to have a record in your computer so that it is easy to go to and update. You can have the information, print out a report, and can easily give that report to all your physicians. There is a form available on my website (www.godrjudy.com) that will at least provide a helpful guideline for listing most of the significant issues in your history and leave you room for adding anything unusual that may not have been covered.

Many people have excellent health, so this history seems rather pointless, but sometimes that information becomes significant down the road. It is amazingly easy to forget things when it's been months or years since it happened and thus not relay them to the doctor. It can also be easy to forget things that bother you from time to time and that might be relevant. Because they aren't bothering you the day you go in for your exam, you may forget about them. It is also easy to forget your history and your medications if you are sick, in pain, or injured. For many healthy people, this history may be less than a page, while for people with significant illnesses, it may take several pages. A listing of significant illnesses in your family members is also important.

Your history should start by having a list of your *current* symptoms (the ones you are visiting the doctor for that day), which can be on a separate piece of paper from your complete history on that Current Complaints Form. Your complete history should start with that basic information on the medications page. It then needs to include, hopefully chronologically and working from the present time backward, all the accidents, injuries, illnesses, surgeries, and significant diagnostic procedures you have had in your life, as well as the results, treatments, and complications. It is also helpful to list medications that you have taken in the past, what they were for, and whether they were helpful, not helpful, or caused problems.

For anything truly significant, you would do well to actually obtain and keep copies of records from doctors, hospitals, labs, X-rays, and any other studies. You are entitled to have a copy of your medical records from any place you receive treatment, including lab and X-ray. When you are having a procedure or treatment, ask what you need to do to get a copy of the records if you don't already know. They may charge you unless it is going directly to your doctor instead of to you.

If you can't get copies, keep a list of the doctors and facilities involved in the treatment. Be aware that doctors are only required to keep records for seven to ten years, and if they move or retire, getting copies can be difficult, so you must be the custodian of your own copy. Obviously, if you have a significant illness or illnesses, this can become a thick bundle of medical records, and you might even want to think of scanning them so you can put them on your computer and be able to give them to your current doctor in a simple format, like a CD, a thumb drive, or the cloud. One of the frustrations that still exist in medicine is being able to get records from one doctor and/or facility to another in prompt fashion, despite all the methods available to expedite that. Hopefully, as electronic medical record systems improve, so will that issue.

Obviously, if you had an uncomplicated appendectomy when you were ten years old in Minnesota and are now eighty and living in California, and there were no problems, that is a simple listing. However, if I had an appendectomy five years ago, and there were complications, and now I am having right lower belly pain again, those records may give some important information that helps the current doctor in assessing and treating me. Unfortunately, medicine is not, never has been, and never will be a simple field where, for example, everyone who has right lower belly pain has appendicitis. Just as a "for instance," that pain can also be from pneumonia, peritonitis, adhesions, an ovarian cyst, a sexually transmitted disease, a pregnancy, diabetes, a hernia, a UTI, and probably at least one hundred other diagnostic entities. Thus, the history you and your records can provide can often help cut this long list down to a short list quickly and effectively to speed up and improve your treatment.

It is also a good idea if you have had, for example, a CT done to assess treatment of a cancer, to have a copy of the report—and possibly even the actual scan—to have available for other doctors who might be involved in treatment. It might prevent the need to have a repeat study, or provide a basis for comparison to see how things are progressing.

Medical Records for Unusual Diseases

Some people have unusual diseases that aren't often seen and usually need to be treated by a specialist. It is usually a good idea to have a copy of records with you about that particular illness which not only provides some of your medical specifics, but it may also contain an article or two about the illness itself. This is especially true if it is one of those strange illnesses that can cause you to suddenly wind up in an ER away from home; failure to have that information could be costly to your well-being. If the doctor doesn't listen to you or believe you, that document can present facts to change their mind. It could also be costly to your and/or your insurance if the ER doctor is trying to investigate somewhat blindly into what is causing your problem, and you are too out of it from your disease to give a useful history and don't have information with you.

With today's technology, you can put your medical information on a flash drive—and there are even some that are small and flat like a credit card—which makes it quick and easy for doctors anywhere with a computer with standard software to look at your information. The day will probably come when that is standard medical practice, and probably you will also be able to opt to have a chip implanted with your medical record, but with all the inconsistencies and incompatibilities that exist in medical record software right now, that day is a long way off. Even though smart phone applications exist now for medical records as well as cloud storage, you still need a hard paper copy that you carry with you that at least briefly gives your most essential information in the event of something, such as an accident that leaves you unconscious or a heart attack or other acute illness that impairs your ability to give information.

6

Things to Do During and After the Visit

Understand Your Doctor's Instructions Before You Leave

B e sure you have talked with the doctor and are clear on what is wanted in terms of tests, medicine changes, disease management and lifestyle changes that you need to carry on after you leave the office. If you are not clear, talk to the doctor, or if that is not an option, talk to the nurse so someone can clarify things for you. Be safe and write things down. That is much more reliable than trusting your memory, especially when you are not feeling good and you may be getting told things you don't really understand.

Learn About Your Illness—and It Won't Be Easy

Once you and your doctor have discussed your illness, the doctor will be a good source of information for you about your disease, what it is, how to manage it, and the lifestyle changes you need to make, as well as some of the places you can turn to for further information. There are many additional ways to learn more about your illness. When warranted, you could also be involved in a support group, either online or live, made up of people with your illness. If you are a book lover, check out your local bookstore, which will often have several good, dependable resources for sale. If the book is just providing you with information and is prepared by a credentialed professional, rather than one selling you Dr. X's wonder cure or bashing the entire medical field, it is more likely to be reliable.

Many people write first-person accounts of their illness. While this is often helpful in many ways, it is important to remember that each person is different. Symptoms, diseases, and treatments vary from person to person. When you have symptoms just like your next-door neighbor or just like the person in a book, it does *not* mean that you have that particular ailment. It is certainly worth bringing up as a consideration, but it is *certainly not* always the right answer. I often recommend specific books for my clients and so do many other doctors. You will do well to check those out first. If funds are limited, the local library can be a great source of information for free.

When using the Internet, it can be even more difficult to determine which resources are good places to turn to and which are not, but there are a few useful things to know. If you have something like cancer or diabetes, national educational organizations like the American Cancer Society (www.cancer.org) or the American Diabetes Association (www.diabetes.org) have a great deal of good information and direct you to other resources. You can Google your disease, but when you do, start with sites sponsored by medical schools or the specialty organizations.

They will provide you with good background information. You can also rely on resources like the National Institutes of Health, the Centers for Disease Control and Prevention (CDC), the National Academy of Sciences, and World Health Organization (WHO). Valuable information can also be gleaned from the websites for the Mayo Clinic and Harvard Medical School. You may want to check out sites from high-quality foreign medical sources that may have a different slant on the illness and treatment options.

Sites like Wikipedia are okay, but they are limited in their scope. Medpagetoday.com really makes a good attempt at being objective, but Medscape and some other sites do have to be viewed cautiously because they do a lot of advertising and some of their "information" is actually advertorial content. Whenever you read something labeled "medical," "holistic," "naturopathic," or anything else around health and wellness, if it seems more like commercial than fact, it probably is. If it is valid, you will find several other places discussing its benefits.

Be very careful. A great deal of information out there is (a) barely disguised advertising for either standard or "alternative" medicine, (b) unfiltered garbage from people with little knowledge and lots of opinion, (c) info from people pushing a special cause, (d) info from people who are "fruitcakes," or (e) even info from people with malicious intent. While I don't want to whitewash the problems in mainstream medicine, there are many other things out there that are driven by malevolence, stupidity, and greed.

When you come across books, websites, and so on where their main intent is to discredit mainstream medicine, especially when they pronounce that they have the magic cure for "disease x that the medical community has been hiding from you," *tread with great caution.* They probably just want to clean out your wallet. Hopefully, their magic treatment will be as benign as vitamins, but you can't count on that, either.

In general, legitimate alternative treatments are used by quite a number of mainstream doctors, although getting your insurance to pay for these alternatives may be an impossible mission. Legitimate alternative-care advocates are generally trying to work in tandem with mainstream medicine to improve quality of care. Those who are less legitimate not only spew venom about the establishment, they also usually have a full line of magical products—which usually are little more than colored water, oils, or vitamins sold at outrageous prices and, often, with no quality control. While I have a great appreciation for vitamins, supplements, herbs, amino acids, and so on (and frequently prescribe useful ones to my patients), the old saying is true: "If it sounds too good to be true, it probably is."

A man in Dallas in the early 1980s worked in a doctor's office as a tech. He had his own side business of "treating" people with his wonderful elixir. It was nothing but an intravenous (IV) of vitamins. For this concoction, he charged $125 and had many people duped into believing he was doing something wonderful. That's a lot of money to pay for the equivalent of a sugar pill, or more correctly, about twenty-five cents' worth of vitamins, even if it helps just like oral vitamins do. He did get put out of business. That is just one example out of thousands. Look at the book flyers you get and the ads you see on the Internet. You will see multitudes of these people peddling their wares every day. If you take more time to read their books or listen to their infomercials, you will soon see they are peddling different magic cures for the same disease at different times.

Sadly, these charlatans make it more difficult for some of the more legitimate natural alternatives, ancient Chinese medicine practices, and so on to get the respect and utilization that might be justified. The effects of these alternative treatments are also usually harder to document. Contrary to what people are led to believe, many physicians are open to the use of almost anything they think will help their patient, whether it is mainstream or not. There is, of course, a wide spectrum of doctors, from those on the cutting edge of science and medicine to those who haven't changed anything they do since they were in residency.

You need to learn to be cautious even about things that come from seemingly credible sources. Medical history is filled with not just the progress that has been made, but the mistaken paths that were followed, and important innovations that were not followed at all, or not for many years (like hand washing). In addition, there has been abundant information from many sources about the importance of emotional wellness as a key factor to the creation of physical wellness, but we don't send everyone who has a medical problem for counseling so they will do better. (Think Dr. Bernie Siegel, Dr. Carl Simonton, and *Laughter Is the Best Medicine*, which all demonstrate the power of the mind to heal the body.) Although mind power helped me recover from a broken hip quickly, I still needed an orthopedic surgeon to stabilize the fracture first.

There are real issues, some of which will be discussed later, of doctors being trained with wrong information, often driven by pharmaceutical and equipment companies in both open and covert fashion. Some physicians out there also have a whole array of their own problems and misinformation. For example, many conscientious parents jumped on the bandwagon of wanting to protect their children from autism, based on information that was overhyped and subsequently proved incorrect, that came basically from *one* physician who claims immunizations caused autism. Thus, their children did not get immunized for diseases like whooping cough and measles. The current result of that is that we have ongoing epidemics of measles and whooping cough.

Just as I was writing this book, I read an online article by a "doctor." He was ranting about how the medical establishment was hiding information from the public about influenza, how it flares up every year, how vaccines don't help based on articles *he* read in medical journals, and how one should not allow these toxins to be injected through an *IV*. When I reviewed his credentials, I could see that he was a chiropractor who doesn't even know that immunizations are given into the *muscle* or by *mouth*, but *not* in the vein. Yet he proclaimed himself an expert about why people shouldn't have immunizations. Chiropractors have their place, but they do not have equivalent training to a medical doctor or a doctor of osteopathic medicine (DO). Some chiropractors *do* refer to themselves as physicians. While I don't see influenza vaccines being as effective as polio vaccines, for example, they are not a source of IV toxins.

You can see the risks in getting information and the difficulties you face. You want to seek information from truly established and presumably credible resources who are supposed to be held to some standard of ethics. What do you think the risks are in getting information from someone has no training and no code of ethics? What good information will you get from those people who have their magic formula product X that is probably not based on any kind of sound information from anywhere? They are just out looking for gullible souls to fill their pocketbook—a modern-day snake oil peddler.

I review some of these sites just to see what they are doing. Recently, I came across one where the doctor was pushing his brand of expensive alternative products. He explained he was no longer licensed and claimed it was because the medical establishment didn't like the way he disagreed with them about his alternative care. What that told me is that he is incompetent, unethical, sexually inappropriate, or chemically addicted, and could not be retrieved—by the best efforts of the medical licensing board—to get him to change his ways. If doctors only had to disagree with the establishment to lose their license, there would be few licensed doctors in this country. Needless to say, it did not convince me to buy his product. I am more concerned about the other doctors who probably should lose their licenses because they make a great deal of money at things like prescription mills. But they can afford lawyers who fight to keep them licensed.

The bottom line is this: You must work to find a healer you trust, based on your experience with them. You need to be able to get information from them. Ask them your questions about given information and where else you might look for comparison facts. Do a lot of comparing yourself—that will help you learn to spot those sources that are doing their best job to present accurate information, and those that are just a platform to sell more snake oil.

Know or Learn about Your Medications

Overview

Clearly, the optimum number of medications to take is zero. While everything else is a compromise, these compromises have done a lot to improve the quality of our lives. Properly used, medications are a great tool to overcome those things we cannot overcome with proper self-care and mind power. Medications are a powerful tool for bad or for good, but just like with a chainsaw, if you don't learn to use them properly, they can do a lot of damage.

Once again, carry that list with you that contains all your essential medical information as was discussed in an earlier chapter. (Go to www.godrjudy.com to download the form.) It is also a good idea to leave copies with family members and a trusted neighbor, especially when you have a lot of medical issues and when you travel. Hopefully, it will never be needed for anything critical, but it definitely will make it much easier for you to be an active, effective participant in your own health care.

There are two important reasons to always carry this information with you. First, you always have it available to show to any doctor when you go to their office. Second, if you are rendered unable to give your history in a medical crisis, an ER doctor, an emergency medical technician (EMT), or paramedic coming to your aid can give you better help more quickly. This simple trick will allow the doctors to continue meds whose absence might be life threatening, and avoid those that could cause a worsening of your problems. If, for example, you list that you are an insulin-dependent diabetic, have seizures, heart disease, or other major issues, that disease will be looked into first as the most-likely cause of your current issue and increase your chance of getting the proper treatment more quickly. When your doctor doesn't have to walk in totally blind to your problems, it is helpful. That little bit of preparation with your information could even save your life.

It is important to list and learn about OTC medications and herbal medicines—as well as prescription medications—because of effects they have that may block, increase, or otherwise modify, the effects of prescription medications that are being taken. They can also sometimes create problems, or kill you, all by themselves. It is always important to look at not only all your medications and their effects and side effects, but also the possible interactions that can happen.

Vitamin E and aspirin, for example, are both OTC medications that can increase the effect of your blood thinners, so that you have more issues with bleeding than is desired. Their presence in your body makes it more difficult to get good control of any bleeding. Some medications might block the effects of another med, while yet another medication might increase the effects of some other medication. Don't get wrapped up in trying to interpret all of this yourself; it requires years of knowing how all this works. Very often, a doctor may use side effects or drug interactions as a positive benefit of combining drugs, rather than something that increases your problems. People often panic when they get a print out from their pharmacy listing some of these *possible* problems. When you read those lists of effects and side effects and interactions remember that only means it *could* happen in someone. It does *not* mean all, or even *any*, of them will occur in you. Do try to get your doctor to research the drug side effects and interactions, but if necessary, go to another resource, such as the pharmacy or available books.

When you get multiple drugs from the same family of drugs, or too high a dose of medication in certain families of drugs, that can be a major problem. For example, the serotonin-based meds for depression are good, but if you take too much because perhaps you have one doctor prescribing one for depression and another doctor prescribing another member of the serotonin family for pain and *another* doctor prescribing a member of the family for weight loss, you can develop an adverse reaction because of the cumulative effects of the three meds, even though each one may be prescribed at a therapeutic dosage. With medicine, like many other things in life, *too much* of a good thing *can turn into a bad thing.* An extreme example of this is that you can drink yourself to death with just wonderful, essential water.

Know What Your Meds Are For

Whenever you are put on a medication, ask what it is for. If you are on more than one medication for something, ask your doctor if you need more than one medication for that disorder. Pay attention to the instructions on your prescription bottle. I find it incredibly frustrating (and it can be dangerous) when I am treating people, and I am trying to get a listing of their medications and they literally have *no idea* of the name, the strength, and so on—much less what they are taking it for. They may know they take "a little white pill" for some unknown reason or that their thyroid pill is "pink," or something equally minimal and unhelpful. If we had only one white pill in the world, it would be no problem, but skim through the picture index of any drug reference text, and you will see literally hundreds of them.

You need to realize this is an important part of *your* health. You need to help your doctor help you. It is generally useful for you to learn at least a little bit about your medications and the things good and bad that they can bring about. However, if you know you are one of those people who are then going to have every problem listed or worry about them excessively, it may be in your best interest not to do that. Generally, an informed patient is a much better patient, and if you have a disorder that is rare, unusual, or requires unusual medications, it is all the more important that you be able to either know more about your disease and your medications for it or at least carry with you documentation about your illness and its treatment provided by other caregivers that you can share with your current physician.

All too often, people take medications without having any idea what they are for. Displaying total trust in the doctor and the pharmacy to give the right medication, means people are taking no responsibility for knowing what they are getting or why they are getting it. They are not double checking to see if the medication is right. It is, unfortunately, also necessary to really know your pharmacy and check to be sure that the pharmacy is dispensing the right medication. I have not only had pharmacies dispense wrong amounts, but also they have dispensed wrong meds and mixed different dosages of the same med in the same bottle—for medications written for me—as a physician. If this happens to me as a physician, you can be sure it happens to you. If it takes the pharmacy and you a few minutes to check things when you pick up your prescription, it is better to ask and to check it out than to wind up with problems from not getting a medicine you need or getting the wrong medication, so your problem isn't resolved. A good pharmacy checks with you about the names of the meds they are refilling and verifies your name and birthdate before they even hand the medication to you.

To learn more about your medications than you are getting from your doctor or your pharmacy, there are some good books available in most bookstores to help you know about both prescription and OTC medications, what they are for, what they look like (if they are name brand), and issues with side effects and interactions. You can also research this on the Internet, but use caution in the sites you choose to pick information from.

A great irony I see too often is the patient who is extremely worried about the side effects of a prescription medication, but he is not worried about the effects of street drugs he consumes, or the alcohol he drinks or the cigarettes he smokes or other ways he abuses his own body.

Be Aware of Medication Effects and Side Effects

You will frequently get verbal information from your doctor and almost always get a printed handout from your pharmacy about your medications. You should read this information about your medications and be familiar with it. Most pharmacists are also quite willing to talk with you about questions or concerns about your meds, and they can be a valuable resource about preventing potential problems and letting you know when to return to your doctor for problems. However, do not *stop* a drug just because there has been a warning about a certain combination of medicines. It might be something as simple as that the combination of the two drugs increases the level in your blood of one or the other or both, and your doctor may be doing that *intentionally* as a more effective way to increase the working amount of the medication in your system. The way to find out is to ask the doctor, even if you need to call the office and relay a message through the staff. Do keep in mind that nowadays pharmaceutical companies *do* go overboard to warn about complications that can arise (as well as make exaggerated claims about their benefits)—to the point where you could get terrified just reading the list. This can also come from pharmacy printouts, which are generated by a computer program that is trying to cover all options and angles.

This is an attempt to include what *might* happen, not just the things that are likely to happen. These instructions are meant to cover the wide range of biological differences in the people the meds are given to and the number of meds that are dispensed. It is also a step to protect against lawsuits. If every patient was identical and responded exactly the same way to any given medicine, life would be much simpler and fewer doctors would be needed. With drugs, foods, plants, animals, water- and airborne chemicals, and anything else that can get on or into your system, each person responds a bit differently. While the problem may have a one in a million chance of happening, if you happen to be that one person, it is a 100 percent problem for you.

The key word here is *possible*. You should be aware of possible side effects and problems. The fact that a problem is on the list does *not* mean it *will* happen. It means it *could* happen in somebody. It is always an important issue to look at, but not always *the* issue. I generally give this advice to my patients: "Anything can happen with any medication or combination of medications, and I am prescribing them to you in a way that hopefully minimizes that risk. If something unusual or possibly bad happens to you after you start a new medicine, call the doctor, and check on it. If you can't reach your doctor promptly, stop the medication until you *can* reach them. If it is a severe reaction, do not waste time calling anyone; just go to the emergency room."

I also try to start only one medicine at time. If you start more than one medicine, you have no idea which one might be giving benefit or causing a problem. This isn't always possible, but it is the ideal way to do things. It does, however, require some patience on your part and the part of the doctor.

Selling Sickness

Those of you who watch a great deal of TV are quite aware of all of the TV advertisements that push medication after medication. The advertisers would be quite happy to have you on *all* of them at the same time, since it would be good for their bottom line. This same excess advertising is found in magazines and in supermarket newspapers. This is *not* advertising aimed at educating the public; it is advertising that is convincing you that you need their product.

An interesting feature of many patients is that even though they may have been developing their medical or mental problems for *years*, they tend to come in wanting a magic wand/instant (which generally doesn't exist) resolution of their problem. People also want to instantly shed the weight they have been gaining over many years. The drug companies play on this personality trait to get people to ask for their magic cures. The snake oil peddlers out there do the same thing. It takes a bit more patience to do things right, but it is—by all means—the safest and the most likely way to improve your health with the fewest possible medications at the lowest possible cost of both money and problems.

Cost Issues

Don't hesitate to mention to your doctor if your medication price is going to be a problem for you. Sometimes, they can give you samples to get you through an illness if the need is temporary. If the need is long term, however, those newer medications, available as free samples, are also the priciest of the meds and are often not significantly better than some meds that have been around longer, are less expensive, and may already be generic.

Also, with the newer drugs, insurance may not pay for them unless you have tried and failed everything that is older and less expensive. The manufacturer will often give doctors coupons that will help reduce the amount of your copay quite a bit. For some people, the cost is still too high, and it is much better to talk with your doctor and find a workable solution than just not take a medication. Not taking a medication can be a bad solution to your problem, and most doctors will work diligently to help you in this area if you just let them know the problem. In addition to doctors modifying what they prescribe, there are also patient assistance programs in place at many pharmaceutical companies. If your income qualifies you, they will provide the medication free or at a reduced cost, usually through your doctor's office.

7

Things to Consider That Can Save You Money

Dealing with Pharmacies

You need to know several things about medications and pharmacies that will help lower your medical care costs and help ensure you are getting the proper medications.

First, you must learn to pharmacy shop by checking with several different pharmacies and checking their prices for the same product. Check the prices for both the generic and the name brand. You will find some pharmacies are reluctant or even downright unwilling to give you that information. Others will hedge with things about your insurance and so on. Insist on the price if you pay cash. If the pharmacy won't give you the price, don't deal with them. You will find as you start checking that the same medication can have a wide range of prices. You will find that the same pill, the same strength, and the same number of pills, may have a price that may vary up to five-fold and more.

A good place to start your check is to go to someplace like Costco (www.costco.com) that has an online listing of their prices. Another website—www.goodrx.com—compares prices for certain prescription drugs at all the pharmacies who sell this medication in your ZIP code. These websites' prices will provide a starting place for your comparison. Since these are the cash-basis prices, your cost should drop further if you have insurance, based on whatever your particular policy chooses to pay on your behalf.

For an even wider comparison base, you may want to check some of the websites, such as the Canadian ones for prescription drugs. Also, unless you have tried the generic version of a medication and it doesn't work for you, ask for the generic. When the doctor writes the name brand of the drug on the prescription blank, even though it is clearly printed on the form that a generic may be substituted, pharmacies will often try to fill it with the higher-priced name-brand drug. I often get a request for a preauthorization for the filling of an expensive name-brand drug, but when we call the pharmacy and remind them they can fill it with generic, the need to go through all the preauthorization paperwork goes away. Why do pharmacies do this? Could it be mostly for the money? Can you blame them for that? Why do insurance companies sometimes pay for the *more expensive* meds rather than the less expensive ones? It's just one of the glitches in the saga of American medical economics.

Second, it is helpful if you can find a pharmacy that is personal enough that they will get to know you and will work with you to get the best possible price if you are having problems affording your meds. Sometimes, the pharmacies (and the doctors' offices) will have coupons on hand that will reduce the amount of copay that you have on some of the newer and older drugs. You may want to talk to the pharmacist as well as your doctor about whether there are older and cheaper drugs that will do the same thing as the newest medication. New medications are always much more expensive than the older medications that they replace. I find it amazing that many drug companies do not reduce the price of their name brand drugs even a little bit once they go generic, much less have a price that comes anywhere close to the price of the generic. Sometimes, the new drug, coming out seven to ten years later, is ten or even thirty times the price of the drug it replaces. This is just for a slight change in the molecule and often little change in how well the medication works.

This is particularly true when they just modify the drug to a slower release-rate form (CR- or XR-type drugs) with no significant change to the drug itself. Even with generics, some pharmacies will charge you little mark up over their cost—especially the larger chains—while others (including some of the other larger chains) will charge you several times their cost for the medication. Even when looking at generics, pharmacy shopping may help your budget.

A third issue in dealing with pharmacies is that they will often tell you they don't have something, don't have enough, or will have to owe you the balance. Occasionally, they just short you on the prescription. This can be a real issue for *you* if you run out early, and the insurance won't fill it, because it is too soon—or the doctor won't rewrite a controlled substance because it is too soon, and so on. You must check the count on your meds soon after you get them.

With a new prescription, it may be good to ask them right away whether they have enough of the medicine to fill your prescription. If they don't, and you can't wait a few days, check with other area pharmacies and consider transferring the prescription. Keep in mind that if a pharmacy chooses to, they can get any medication, unless it is in short supply in the market generally, within twenty-four hours from the pharmaceutical warehouses, although most of them understandably prefer ordering on a weekly basis. If they can't fill your medication when you need it, be sure you ask things like: Do you have it in a generic? When can you get it in? Does one of your other stores have it? Does one of your competitors carry it? They usually won't answer that last question, but *you* can call around and check with other pharmacies before you give the okay to fill with a given pharmacy. Sometimes, your doctor will have samples to cover you for a few days. Insurance companies are causing some problems for some people by making them use particular pharmacies so that changing drug stores isn't an option, but usually you still have some choices. Insurance companies also provide mail-in service for maintenance medications. This option may actually be a good deal because they mail you a ninety-day supply of medication; your copay is lower; and, often, they will send you a reminder when a refill is due.

Fourth, when you take a script in, be sure the pharmacy is going to fill it for you fully and within a specified time or take it to a different pharmacy. If it isn't urgent to have it filled the day you planned to pick it up, you can even consider leaving the partial script there until they can fill it fully. Obviously, if you really know the folks at your pharmacy, this isn't an issue. One important way for you to avoid some of these problems is to request your refill a few days ahead rather than calling it in the day you take your last pill and expect it to be ready that night. If you have medications that are unusual or are controlled substances that might not be as readily available, let your pharmacy know. They will usually respond well to being asked to keep some on hand for you around whatever time of month you usually need a refill of your medication. In that same line, if a refill will need approval from a doctor's office, you should know that doctors have many things to take care of during the course of a day. Stopping in the middle of other urgent tasks to fill someone's prescription request the moment it comes in is not realistic. Always allow at least a day. Do not call on Friday or Saturday unless you won't need the med until Monday or Tuesday. Know that sometimes when you call the pharmacy for a refill, and they say they have sent the request to the doctor, they *have not*. With the hundreds of scripts some of them fill in a given day, things can get mixed around a bit. You may need to contact the doctor's office yourself.

The fifth issue is the whole complex of interactions between the pharmacy and the insurance company. You are well-advised to check ahead of time to find out what your insurance company will pay for and how much and which generics are acceptable, and so forth. Doing this can prevent you from having to pay full price for something when the insurance is also paying. Doing this will also keep your copay where it belongs or inform you that you will have to pay full price because your insurance won't cover it.

Another interesting trick I just became aware of is really underhanded. Now, you might have an insurance copay that is higher than the *cash price*. Another difficult issue is that while insurance may pay for IV meds you might get via something like home health, they apparently don't pay for the equipment that is needed to give the medication IV, leaving you stuck with that cost. It seems like a bit of a shell game, but forewarned is forearmed. Know how to look out for yourself in the pharmacy/insurance reimbursement arena.

Understanding Diagnostic Testing: When You Need It, When You Don't, and How to Get Some of It Done With Less Expense

General Information

By diagnostic testing, I am referring to the tests you get done to help diagnose your medical issues, including blood tests, urine tests, X-ray (radiology), CT Scans, MRIs, mammography, lung function tests, biopsies, colonoscopies, allergy testing, psychological testing, and so on. It is important for you to understand that diagnostic testing simply reflects what is going on in your body *at that moment*. It can change fairly quickly in any direction, depending on what is happening to you. One of the closest analogies is that it is a lot like taking your temperature, which can change because of a number of things—some which are important and some which are not. If you are running a fever when you have pneumonia that does not mean you *always* run that high temperature. Temperature is a test that reflects what is going on right then.

Ideally, doctors perform testing for three basic reasons: (a) they may order certain clusters of tests as screening tests employed in routine health exams just to be sure nothing is abnormal that would signal an early disease processes, (b) they might order some specific tests that they feel will help confirm or deny the presence of certain medical problems they are evaluating you for, or (c) they order tests to follow the course of a disease or the results of treatment.

When there was more pressure of a threat of malpractice suits in prior years, some doctors would order a wide array of tests just to be sure they didn't miss anything so they wouldn't be sued. That put patients through quite a bit and cost a lot for both the patient and the insurance company. Fortunately, that is not as much of an issue any more.

Unfortunately, insurance companies often make it more difficult to get needed testing done because they don't want to pay for it, causing doctors to have to do extra work (and you can help with this process[2]) to get it approved. There have also been tests, such as mammograms and prostate-specific antigen (PSA) testing, which were religiously performed on a regular basis as screening tests because the belief—at the time—was

---

2   When insurance denies testing that the doctor feels is important, contact more than just the insurance company directly to complain. Don't be afraid to go up the chain of command. Talk to the human relations department at your employer, and let them put a little pressure on the insurance company, also. Your employer needs to know when an insurer isn't delivering on the contract properly. I have known people *employed by their insurance carrier* who still had to go through some heated battles and go up the line with their insurer to get urgent testing done. You may need to go to supervisors and, sometimes, to a vice president in charge of claims with your insurer to get needed attention.

that they were necessary to help detect disease early. Currently, evidence is emerging that, for much of the population, doing those tests every year is not only unnecessary, but it may cause some unnecessary treatments, in the case of prostate, and be of little benefit at that frequency for breast cancer (unless you have a family history) as examples.

Diagnostic testing, along with everything else in medicine, is constantly changing as we learn more and more over time and as new techniques and new studies come along.

One of the latest hot topics is genome testing to help direct diagnosis and treatment, but this is in its early stages. Only time will tell how helpful it becomes. In my forty years of being in the medical field, I have seen many treatments, tests, and medications go from "hot" to "not-so-hot" and even be totally phased out.

Clinical Pathology Labs

Once your doctor has made a diagnosis for you, unless you have a specific medical illness that requires close lab monitoring, such as diabetes, or a medication level that needs to be monitored (like lithium or Depakote), checking your blood-clotting tests when you are on an anticoagulant (blood-thinning) medication (or some other illness where much testing is needed to evaluate or manage a disease), frequent lab work is generally not necessary. Blood and urine screening studies tend to get done along with your annual physical, but usually you don't need testing in between unless an illness arises. Generally, any time someone goes into a hospital, however, he will have labs done even if he was discharged just two days earlier and is back again. There is no reason to suspect changes in lab values, but just when you are *sure* nothing could have changed, it will have.

Lab errors do happen. If there is something on a lab test result that does not match with how you know things should be, let your doctor know. I have had things happen at a hospital such as a lithium level on a patient suddenly dropping. Having first trained as a pathologist, my inclination is to check other charts and, if it is happening in all the patients, let the lab and the other doctors know there is an ongoing lab problem. If it isn't happening elsewhere, then I know I need to look further into what is wrong with the patient. When in doubt, have your doctor check it out.

Basic Test Purposes

A *urinalysis* is a test that looks primarily for evidence of a UTI, kidney disease, urinary tract bleeding, diabetes, overhydration or dehydration, pregnancy screening, and drug abuse. Not all these things are necessarily screened for each time. Despite one of my patients recently insisting that her doctor did a urine test and diagnosed her with a stomach ulcer, that is *not* one of the purposes of that test—not even close!

A *screening blood chemistry test* usually looks at those chemicals in the blood that indicate things are, or are not, functioning like they should. It checks the electrolytes (sodium, potassium, and chloride), your sugar, cholesterol and other lipid levels, and any abnormalities in the function of your kidneys and liver. It is not at all unusual to also check thyroid-function screening tests. Other tests are ordered based on suspected illnesses, to check the status of your medication, or to check for alcohol or other drugs. They should not, however, be performed too frequently just as a screening test. It isn't necessary and doesn't really give any new information and runs up the cost of your care. If a doctor wants to check your serotonin level to see if you are depressed, that is not a valid test. A lithium level is only meaningful if you are taking lithium as a medication. It is of no value to diagnose bipolar disorder.

A *complete blood count (CBC)* is done to look for evidence of infection, anemia, other blood diseases like leukemia, and whether you are putting out enough of each of the blood cell types. Generally, if it is normal with the annual screening, it isn't needed again for a while, unless there is a new problem.

Most laboratory tests are not tremendously expensive for the lab. In fact, it is inexpensive for the lab to run all the tests together as a panel. The lab, the hospital, or the ER, however, tends to bill you and/or the insurance for each test separately at a much higher cost rather than as a package cost.

Why Medicare in its wisdom wanted them billed separately (unbundled) instead of together is beyond my comprehension!

The technology that led to all the automated lab tests allows a whole panel of tests to be performed at the same time on the same specimen. It no longer requires intensive time from the staff to perform one test type at a time the way it did forty years ago.

These basic tests can be augmented with any number of other specific tests both to diagnose your disease and to manage the course of treatment. Just listing all of them would probably take several more pages of text and be quite boring for you.

Laboratory studies will vary in cost from one facility to another. If you have lab studies you need done and are not hospitalized, you might want to call around and see who has the best prices. Generally, for lab or X-ray, you probably want to use a free-standing facility rather than a hospital, if possible, since there can be a several-fold difference in the price—just like with the pharmacies. This is particularly an issue if you are paying cash, but it can also make a marked difference in your copay.

Radiology Studies

Radiology has advanced incredibly in the last forty years and we now have many techniques available to help diagnose and guide treatment of disease. In addition to regular X-rays, CT scans are a much more sophisticated way of doing sequential X-rays through the body, rather than one study that shows everything in less detail. We also have the

MRI which uses a magnetic field technology to study what is happening in the body. We have gone from technology that could only allow us see broken bones and big problems, such as tumors and infection, to technology that can study abnormalities a few millimeters in size in the body easily. There is even some technology now that helps assess how an organ is functioning, rather than just how it looks.

The rule of thumb is to start with the simpler (and less expensive) technology and only go to the more complex ones if you *need* that to get closer to the answer. What is important to you as a consumer is that you don't want to be going out and getting multiple X-rays and CT scans unless it is necessary because of the cumulative exposure to radiation and the cost. Thus, if you have had a recent study and are now somewhere else, and they want to repeat the same study, see if they can use the one that was previously done. Whenever possible, have a copy of the report, which will also give a file number that may allow the doctor to access the raw data to evaluate independently if the written report didn't answer the questions. Sometimes, it is appropriate to repeat, but let your doctor know there was a prior study. It may eliminate that need. In addition, when dealing with things like suspected cancer, infection, or even a fracture, having different images to compare across a span of time can be helpful to determine diagnosis, prognosis, or progression of disease or its healing.

The other take-away message for you about radiology studies is that the same study may have a different price tag in one place compared to another. Obviously, if you are in a hospital, you will have to do the studies there, but—given a choice between a hospital-based radiology test and the same thing being done in a free-standing outpatient facility—may reflect a dramatic difference in price. A test may cost $2,400 in the hospital facility and $600 in the free-standing facility. Also, it is often easier and quicker to get the testing in the free-standing facility. This is a point when it may be well worth your time to shop prices.

Do realize that errors can also happen in radiology, so if something doesn't seem right, get it checked out. I had a recent psychiatric inpatient who went to the ER complaining of belly pain and swelling. He did have an abdominal film. It was read as normal, and he was sent to the psychiatric unit. When our internist checked him and then read the X-ray himself, he found that the man had a serious fecal impaction. It was amazing how much better he felt when the real problem was finally diagnosed and treated.

The High Cost of Medical Care and What You Can Do About It

While there may be some positive aspects for medical care being a major part of the economic system of this or any other country, that big cost gets spread out to all of us in a variety of ways that cut into our personal income. As I mentioned previously, in our country, medical care accounts for 17 percent of the total annual federal budget. This only includes the components for Medicare, Medicaid, Veterans Administration, Military Medical Care, Tricare, and Champus. This increases your taxes, but it doesn't include all the outlay by the private sector, including your out-of-pocket costs. When you add in all the varying components that go into medical care and supporting the medical care industry, it is probably the largest employment sector and income generator in the country. There is the cost of your copay, OTC, uncovered treatments, costs in time missed from work for being sick, lost wages from being sick, the less obvious tax for Medicare, the cost of your insurance, taxes on cigarettes and alcohol to help offset the costs of related illnesses, things like hospital district taxes that are a part of your property tax, and on and on.

Because people are doing less to prevent and/or to properly manage their health problems, more has to be spent to diagnose and treat them. With the onset of Obamacare, there is now much more of a push for preventive medicine—a long overdue improvement. Had insurance companies been vested in the best interests of the population as a whole, this would have been put in place long ago. If we could ever find a way to make preventive medicine as financially attractive as selling illness, we could solve the problem. Understanding these issues is a step in the right direction.

Become a Knowledgeable Consumer of Medical Services

The purpose here is to help you understand the high cost of medical care and what things you can do to make it more reasonable for yourself and to begin to give yourself a healthier lifestyle—so you don't *need* all that care.

One of the worst offenses on the part of *some* patients is their refusal to take good care of their own health, resulting in many doctor visits and hospitalizations that would not be needed if they would just care for themselves better. This care can be as simple as monitoring your blood pressure or your blood sugar, taking your medication regularly, following special diets when they are needed, avoiding excessive eating, not abusing cigarettes, alcohol or drugs (be they street drugs or prescription drugs), or engaging in high-risk behaviors, such as sharing needles, having unprotected sex with relative strangers, driving like you think you are an Indianapolis 500 race driver, riding your motorcycle without a helmet, driving under the influence of chemicals that blur your awareness, etc.

Health care has the *appearance* of being free, because it is paid for by insurance. As a result, people have quit being conscientious consumers of medical care and products. Sadly, many medical components have conspired to make it more difficult for people to know what they are getting and what it will cost. The various entities make it difficult for you to be an informed consumer. While this is partly based on the reality of each disease being different with each person, it is mostly to keep things deliberately vague. Patients tend to have little idea what a visit, a procedure, a medicine or anything else costs until after they have the service and get the bill. This is an issue consumer advocate groups need to address. Stephen Brill's article "Bitter Pill: Why Medical Bills Are Killing Us" in *Time* delineated some of these areas well.

Many people also tend to give little care and attention to the maintenance work they should be doing on their own bodies. When people have an automobile, if they are *responsible* owners, they quickly learn how much it costs to get something fixed, and they also learn how they can prevent a high cost by doing proper maintenance. They also know that *they* have to pay the cost of fixing it. With their bodies, people generally have no idea how much anything costs so they have too little motivation to do the preventive maintenance that keeps them happy, healthy, and in minimal need of medical care.

At a point when health quality should be at an all-time high because of all the available diagnostic tests and improved treatments, it is nowhere near that because people don't care for their own bodies and their own health as well as they care for their cars—*or* their pets. People do not put in place their own "insurance" to give themselves the best health quality they can maintain by taking care of the basic issues totally under their own control. A patient becomes unhappy when the doctors *cannot* give a magic pill (or wave a magic wand) to fix an illness *immediately*—an illness that she has been developing for some time. Using the same automobile analogy, if you abuse your car for years by rarely changing the oil, not putting water in the radiator, and doing body damage so the vehicle is barely running, you wouldn't expect to have your car in the shop for fifteen minutes and have it fixed.

Yet, that is almost how absurd some people's expectations are about how their bodies should be healed. People tend not to want to put *any* effort in to do the needed maintenance work on their bodies or resolve issues that further damage their bodies, such as bad eating habits, excess weight, inadequate exercise, smoking, drug and alcohol abuse, and environmental pollution. They want a magic wand for that also. The magic wand for some is a diet program, a gastric bypass, an electronic cigarette, a short-term rehab, etc. These solutions do not perform magic either.

8

Other Financial Issues
That Can Help You

How It Used To Be

Many people think that because they have insurance, getting medical care should be easy and cost them little. They believe the doctors are raking in the money, because the patient has insurance. In fact, even twenty years ago when doctors got a bigger part of the medical monies than they do currently, they only accounted for 2 percent of the total cost of medical care. It is probably a smaller percentage now. There also *was* a time when dealing with insurance companies and getting the care you needed was straightforward and easy. That time went away with the birth of "managed care" (also lovingly referred to as "mangled care"), which was quickly shown to be a boon to insurance companies and a disaster for the insured and the employers who paid for the insurance.

When I first started practice in 1980, after I performed a service, I (or my staff) simply billed the insurance company, and I promptly got paid at a good rate that covered most of my fee.

That time is gone!

I also recall that when my grandmother was alive and working, she had two insurance policies, and both policies would pay. If the combined payment was more than the bill, she got to keep the difference. That time is *really* gone.

Today, the combined policies will only pay the "allowed" (by the insurance companies) percentage of the bill, you pay the "allowed" copay (or your secondary insurance does), and the doctor is "allowed" to write off the rest. The only way around that system for the doctor now is to only accept direct payment from the patient and to give them the form so they can collect the "allowed" amount from the insurance company and bear the cost of the difference. In the past, insurance paid most of the bill without argument; now it is a serious struggle to collect 25–50 percent of the fee, no matter how reasonable it may be.

In the past, there were no issues with having to get approval from the insurance company before a procedure could be done or a prescription for a certain medication could be written and expect to be filled. The insurance company didn't have to agree ahead of time that the person needed to be hospitalized or operated on or have certain tests done. Unless a doctor's fee was truly outrageous, most charges were paid by the insurance company. It not only hasn't been that way for about twenty years now, but things are getting steadily worse.

For those of you who think the insurance company is your friend, I would recommend you watch Michael Moore's 2007 documentary *Sicko*, which shows quite clearly some of the issues with insurance companies. Of course, there are issues beyond just the insurance companies that contribute to the problems. Those issues also include the doctors, the hospitals, the pharmacies, the pharmaceutical companies, the medical equipment companies, the rip-off artists, and crooks. You, the patient, are included.

Keep in mind that the major financial players in the Medical Industrial Complex consist of the insurance companies, hospitals, pharmaceutical companies, pharmacies, nursing homes, home health care groups, and medical equipment companies. They are interested in your *physical* health only to the extent that it helps their *financial* health. In fact, the more diseased you are, the healthier their finances become.

Know the Issues with Insurance Companies

Since I started practice, events have changed dramatically. Insurance, costing more and more, is demanding more and more from providers— and often more effort from you as a patient. It pays less and less, often using marginal criteria for denying care and/or payment. In this day and age, the *insurance companies*—not the government—dictate what your doctor, hospital, and pharmacy get paid. It's the *insurance companies* who determine what you are "entitled" to be treated for under your insurance, and what treatments they will or will not pay for—whether it is a diagnostic procedure, a treatment procedure, or a medication.

It is not at all unusual for them to *initially* approve something and then say they didn't, when it comes time to pay. If you have a second insurance, it will pay just the copayment, and that combination will generally pay the providers considerably less than what they charge (whether reasonable or not) and that tends to be a relatively fixed fee for most procedures. Your policy may say that it pays "X percent of usual and customary," but the bottom line is they usually pay the same amount no matter what your policy says, and the only way to determine that amount is to look at your explanation of benefits (EOB)—after they pay their part of the bill. That EOB may not arrive in your mailbox for many weeks after the illness, which only adds to the confusion.

Neither you nor the doctor's office is likely to be able to get an answer ahead of time about what the insurance will pay or what your copay is. Although most people don't realize it, *private* insurance—which you pay so dearly for—usually pays only a little bit more than Medicare. (And Medicare, by the way, is *not* free insurance. The premium is paid out of your Social Security, which is also not a free government handout. The Social Security that you receive is based on regular deductions taken from your wages all through your working life. You also have a payroll deduction for Medicare during your working life.) Not only do the private insurance companies pay only a little more than Medicare, they *demand much* more. Part of these demands are in terms of what you have to do to get a procedure authorized, the hoops you have to jump through for the ongoing care, the struggle with them to get the money once you send them the bill. They also want to minimize your treatments to almost nothing. Your secondary insurance is equally as unlikely to pay for a needed treatment as your primary insurance, with rare exceptions. They mainly pick up the copay and the beginning-of-the-year deductibles. Clearly, much of this problem is a result of desire for excess profit on the part of the insurance companies.

Insurance companies will routinely also find ways to delay payments to doctors and hospitals as long as possible. This tactic is used for several reasons. First, if they deny a claim, they are hopeful the doctor's office will not catch the problem, will overlook it, or give up and then *the insurance company* gets to keep all the money, while you get dunned for the bill repeatedly—or the doctor has to "eat it." Second, the longer they keep the money in the bank, the more interest they make on the money, which they put into their profit column. This has been a severe enough problem that laws have been passed to make insurance companies pay doctors timely. Payments must be made within a three-week time frame, but the insurance companies are clever at constructing loopholes, glitches, rule changes, and other ways to keep the money longer. They are successful enough at it that it is more than worth the occasional time they get caught and have to pay a fine. (For a perspective, they make enough from this so that they can tolerate fines in the neighborhood of several million dollars.)

It is good that health care reform has mandated that insurance companies must pay 80 percent of what they collect in premiums on patient care, but I have total faith in the ability of the insurance companies to keep books in such a way that they actually spend less than that—*and* with the amounts of money they collect, they have options for investing the money at high rates of return to kick their ultimate profit even higher. (That profit doesn't get calculated into the monies mandated to go toward benefits.)

Sadly, having insurance has gone from a great benefit which readily paid for needed care, to a system which charges enormous amounts of money while the insurance company makes it more difficult for people to get the benefits they—and their employers—paid for. I have watched this decline happen progressively over my lifetime. In parallel, I have watched patients do less to care for themselves properly and more to misuse the system.

What does the above mean to you as a patient? First, it means someone other than your doctor is in charge of what treatment you will be allowed to get. (P.S. It is *not* the government; it's the insurance company.) Second, it adds to the whole issue of burdening doctors to the point that many limit their treatment to certain insurance, or they will make you pay cash upfront and collect from the insurance company yourself. Third, many doctors won't treat you at all if you have Medicaid or Medicare.

I have had friends who at some point worked for insurance companies in the process of reviewing whether someone got treatment, and they wound up quitting. Why? Because they couldn't stand to be working at a job where they had to deny people treatment for something they needed and were entitled to get under their insurance plan. I've also dealt with many people who have worked for insurance companies and have described some of the things the insurance companies do to keep an unfair share of the money in *their* pocket.

Preventive Tactics to Use with Insurance Companies

What you need to do to defend yourselves in dealing with an insurance company — and this includes *any* insurance company selling insurance for *anything* (be it health, fire, homeowners, automobile, business, and so on)—includes checking the reputation of the salesperson and the company. Analyze and scrutinize the fine print for what you are really getting in your policy. Often, there are many exclusions that you might not even expect in a policy, so you must check carefully to see exactly what is included. Be aware that they do this to businesses and business owners as well as to individuals. This is especially true for medical care. Also, consider the cases of the homeowners who didn't realize they didn't have flood insurance or something of that nature until they needed it. I have seen companies who got insurance for their employees who thought—based on what they were told—that they were providing good benefits to their employees and themselves. They found out later, however, that when they needed the care, the fine print excluded a service they needed.

Most people are aware that dental services and eyeglasses are often not covered. Many policies also either don't provide or severely limit mental health services, despite local and federal law mandating that it be given coverage just like other medical illnesses and not be subject to exclusion or ridiculously low lifetime limits. (The first attempt at what has been called "mental health parity" began about twenty years ago, and it only took effect a few years ago. *That* is another story in itself.)

Another area that is often a problem is the constantly shifting definition of "pre-existing condition." We have had to deal with patients whose insurance denied coverage because the illness was "pre-existing" when, in fact, they had never been treated for anything similar before, much less within the usual one year window of exclusion for "pre-existing." This problem is supposed to be going away under Health Care Reform.

While I believe insurance is a valuable tool which people should use, it can be and is, managed in deceptive ways all too often. They have ways of managing the data to hold on to monies in ways people generally wouldn't even imagine. There are also always some extremely corrupt, fly-by-night insurance companies that pop up and focus on things like scamming seniors out of their savings for worthless insurance. Although they often get caught, it is usually too late for those people who have already been ripped off.

Tricks Insurance Companies Use to Keep from Paying

One of the most common tricks to avoid payment is to give verbal approval for a procedure or admission or something, and then later deny that approval for a wide variety of reasons. This can be anything—you didn't really call them; they didn't really approve it; the person you talked to wasn't authorized; they looked back and that procedure wasn't covered after all; nobody communicated it to them; and so on. I have even seen things as outrageous as that they approve someone's treatment, pay for it, and then *a few months after the patient died* (from an unrelated issue) demand their money back, saying the service wasn't covered. Normally, when they deny something *after* the fact like this, they at least leave you some window for recovering from the patient, but I thought trying to do a "take back" after the patient had died was really sinking to a new low standard in the industry.

Other common tricks have to do with the billing process and can be issues as simple as changing what data needs to be in which box on the form—but not communicating this ahead of time, of course. Medicare did this when the National Provider ID numbers came out and kept changing where the number should go and stalled payments for about six months. Companies will deny they have received the claim. You might think that would be difficult to do in the electronic age, but apparently they have a lot of cyberspace detours that they utilize. They will deny claims for not being filed "timely," even though you have a documented trail of transmission to them. While that time frame is usually a reasonable year, it can be as short as ninety days. There are myriad other ways they will find to reject or to deny a claim, which means you have to determine what they want and refile it. What they are really hoping is that you will overlook it, and— at worst — they will collect extra investment income from that money while it sits in their account.

One of the newest gimmicks is really sneaky. The office files a claim. When they respond, either with payment or denial or some of both, they don't send an EOB to the provider either electronically or by mail. Once a check has dropped into the bank, the staff then has to go winding through a maze of different sites for the provider to finally find the EOB to determine what has and hasn't been paid. And guess what? If it was only denials and there was no check, then unless the office manager is really aggressive and tuned in, they just managed to steal the provider's money —and leave them no recourse to collect from the patient because they "didn't file timely," or didn't refile or didn't make the corrections or whatever. While I am a basically trusting person and like to believe the best of everyone, these kinds of maneuvers get to the point where there is no conclusion to reach other than deliberate deception and manipulation. You must always be on guard and checking with your doctor and your insurance to stay on top of things. Why do *you* need to check also? Because it is your health, your insurance, and your care that will wind up going to a "cash up front only" basis if this kind of situation continues to worsen, and then you will be left to deal with these folks all on your own.

Dealing with Insurance Companies as the Consumer

Always call your insurance company *yourself* before seeing a doctor for the first time. Be sure and ask for benefits relating specifically to the reason that you need to see that particular physician. Ask if that specialty is a covered service, if the physician is in-network, and will they apply a copay, coinsurance, or deductible to the service. Is an authorization required, or is there a visit maximum? When you call the insurance company, demand that they speak to you in layman's terms or ask them to explain things so that you understand them. Each and every time you call insurance companies remember to document the date, time, and name of the person you spoke to (ask for spelling if necessary) and ask for a call reference number. Most insurance companies require the calls to be recorded and documented with a call reference number. Do not be afraid to ask for a manager or supervisor if you can't understand or do not agree with what you are being told. Write down as much of the conversation as you can.

Your insurance company is required to provide you with a copy of an EOB for each claim it receives. It is helpful for you to study these documents carefully; this will help you tremendously with understanding your benefits. A copy of this document will be sent to your physician or other provider as well. The EOB will tell you how much has been paid on your claim and how much you owe for the service. If you paid some or all up front for that particular service, you can subtract that amount from the total that is indicated as your part to pay.

Be aware, however, that some claims or procedures may have multiple bills related to them. These include such charges as lab fees, radiology fees, facility fees, and many other fees—especially if you are treated for inpatient or outpatient hospital services. If you are hospitalized, all the doctors' charges are billed completely separately and are one more issue for you to deal with. When you look at these EOB forms, you will also be able to see how much the doctor or other provider had to write-off.

If you feel that the insurance company did not pay your claim correctly, you may always call or write them with your dispute. It is a good idea to have your EOB available when you are talking to them and even the benefits guide that your employer gave you. I have persuaded insurance representatives to change or override decisions numerous times. In each case, however, I was prepared with details from prior conversations or information confirming my version of the dispute. Sometimes, when a claim was reevaluated, it was because I pled the case of common sense. If you have a valid argument, there is always the possibility that you can get your claim paid; someone on the inside has the authority to make changes if he desires to do so. In the case that you cannot agree with the decision the insurance company has made in reference to your claim or do not feel the insurance company is treating you fairly, you can always get in touch with your human resources (HR) manager who can verify whether the claim was payable or not. The HR manager may well find another insurance company to take over the benefits of the corporation if she is getting numerous complaints about high out-of-pocket costs, inadequate service, or has too many employees who are unhappy with the current plan.

Obamacare

The Health Care Reform Act is a first step in trying to improve the medical care delivery system without having to go to socialized medicine. Although people have run around screaming and in a panic, it will be like much other legislation. Once something like this is put in place, some parts are acted on; some parts are challenged; and some parts get lost somewhere in the halls of government. I find it interesting the amount of screaming the insurance companies have done when they were *included* in the planning. To me, that seems a bit like setting the fox to guard the henhouse!

Some really good aspects that are already in place include the push for *preventive care,* rather than only managing sickness, the inclusion of young people on their parents' insurance until they are twenty six, the elimination of caps for payments, the hopeful elimination of the pre-existing condition exclusion, and the limits on the amount of money insurance companies can direct somewhere *other* than patient care. There is also a bit more help from the federal government to help fund state Medicaid programs.

I see articles about topics like the doctor shortage we will have once there are 30 million more people covered by insurance. Those authors apparently don't realize these same people currently get treated by abusing the system and using up ER space and other venues where they can avoid paying, so taxpayers get to pick up the tab.

I also see large corporations blaming Obamacare for why they have to cut so many of their employees back to part-time and to cut their benefits. My opinion, however, is that they are just using that as an excuse to do the same thing that corporations like Walmart have done for a long time just for that purpose—long before Obamacare was even dreamed of.

Like any major reform, it will be cussed, discussed, stalled, modified, and impeded where possible by those who are more interested in their pocketbooks than anything else. It is a start in the right direction.

Only time will tell where it winds up. My guess, however, is that despite Obamacare or any other attempt to correct the system, the greed of the Medical Industrial Complex will ultimately cause its collapse and a default to socialized medicine.

Other Financial Aspects of Medical Care

From my perspective as a physician, it is frustrating to have to jump through the hoops of the insurance companies, and—sometimes—overly enthusiastic credentialing agencies such as the Joint Commission to do the thing I know how to do, which is to take care of patients. Quite often, it feels more like treating charts than treating patients, especially in the hospital, and it gets increasingly frustrating over time. This is one reason you find more doctors making changes in their medical practices and billing practices. Sometimes they get so frustrated they quit practicing medicine when they could practice for many more years, if these issues had not emerged to make practice so much less emotionally rewarding and enjoyable than it used to be.

Doctors

Doctors are bright about learning what they are taught about medicine, but many of them are truly dumb about business, economics, and politics. They are too busy running on the hamster wheel of medical practice to step back and see or *analyze* what is happening. While most doctors are truly motivated, caring people who try to do what is right for the patient to the best of their ability, there has always been a small percentage of doctors who have done too many procedures that are not justified or charged outrageously for them, or even charged for procedures they didn't perform. There have been those who have been unethical in taking perks from various kinds of vendors, much like members of Congress who have been alleged to take perks from lobbyists.

Even infrequent reading of newspapers past and present reveals some of the scams that have been run by doctors, and the scams sometimes include pharmacies, medical equipment supply companies, referral sources, and so on. Sometimes, it is for rendering services through multiple clinics at once or sending people out to recruit patients—or at least their critical information—to bill for services that are never rendered. The pill mills that have dispensed such enormous amounts of abusable prescription drugs are usually abusing the insurance system as well as abusing the patients by giving them way too much medication. These overprescribed patients can either abuse it themselves, or they may sell it on the street and damage still more people.

Although most people who go to medical school are honest and well-motivated, some—just like in any other profession—are a disgrace to the profession. Sadly, they often make much more money than honest doctors and then are good at hiring expensive lawyers who will defend them. Whenever you have any questions about the ethics of a doctor, checking with the state medical licensing board is a good place to start. You might even find the information just checking on line.

If you spend much time in a community, you can begin to get a sense of which doctors and hospitals are of higher quality and more ethical (as well as the opposite). More significantly, those people who are into getting excessive amounts of abusable prescription drugs from physicians rapidly learn by word-of-mouth (and so do physicians by being alert about their patient's behaviors) which doctors are the ones to go to who will basically give you anything you want, whether it is indicated or not, and whether it is abusable or not (the "candy doctors"). It sometimes takes a bit longer to ferret out those who are incompetent, unethical, or immoral in other ways. Generally efforts are ongoing in every state to clean out undesirable doctors and to retrieve those who can be helped.

Hospitals

Hospitals, fortunately, have changed a great deal from their original intent, which was to be a place for people to go to die. In more recent history, they became a place to isolate those with infections like leprosy and tuberculosis from the rest of the population, as well as a place to contain those who were too impaired either physically or mentally from their illnesses, both to provide them some comfort and to spare others from having to look at or deal with them.

Hospitals are now associated with the struggle to overcome illness and to stay alive (be that mentally, physically, or both) or to bring new life into the world. Unfortunately, statistics that suggest 100,000 to 200,000 people a year die in hospitals from needless mistakes, while about a million a year have some kind of hospital care–induced problem, raise concerns that they seem to be returning to the role of "a place to die" for too many people.

Many *medical* illnesses used to result in "insanity" that continued to exist until the person died from that illness. Many of these are ailments that we now treat and often cure before they get to the point of causing rampant and untreatable mental illness or even serious medical illness. This includes things like brain tumors, strokes, infections of the brain, endocrine diseases like goiter and Cushing's disease, cancer, seizures, etc. There is an extremely wide range of medical problems that can and, when left untreated, do result in mental illness that used to be handled by just putting people away in the asylums to die. These were people stuck away in the hospitals of even one hundred years or so ago.

As we have learned about simple things like washing our hands to prevent the spread of disease between patients (which is sadly still an ongoing struggle to get people to do), learned more about surgery and the prevention of infections, and developed medications that treat infections and other illnesses, hospitals have become a place for people to go with more serious illnesses to be diagnosed and treated in ways that couldn't even be imagined one hundred years ago.

With the development of better ways to do things, and the advent of marketing, there are many positive things that can now be done in the hospital that save people's lives. Surgical technology has improved some things to the point that they can now be done as outpatient surgery, with the person in the hospital less than twenty-four hours from start to finish. While this is great in the eyes of the insurance companies for limiting costs, and even greater for the patient who doesn't have to be laid up as long, out of work as long, or put as at-risk for hospital-acquired disease, it is "bad" for the hospitals who want to keep their beds filled, their staff working, and their profits flowing in.

Sometimes, there are some slips in quality of care because the staff is underpaid or undertrained and that may result in complications, such as exposure to infections and other careless mistakes. Sometimes, there is a tendency to want to keep patients too long—or to charge too much. This whole system sets up a series of checks and balances between hospital and insurance, but in the middle, it tends to be the patients, and sometimes the doctors, who get squeezed.

There was an interesting commentary on a medical site (medpagetoday.com) recently that hospitals are actually adversely affected by having a lower rate of complications in surgical procedures. This is because when there are complications, there are additional days in the hospital and extra charges for those services. The system set up for payments is supposed to limit the length of treatment for any given illness based on the number of days it *should* take to get someone well. Complications allow for additional codes and charges. It is difficult to find a perfect solution.

There is no doubt in my mind that hospitals, insurance companies, pharmaceutical companies, and equipment supply companies are all involved in a financial shell game where each increases their prices and blames the others for the need to do so. It is also clear that when a hospital charges for a procedure or service, there will almost always be add-ons. Steven Brill's article "Bitter Pill: Why Medical Bills Are Killing Us" in *Time* clearly covered some of these issues.

My sister also had an experience with a hospital trying to collect more money than the insurance company had allowed. The hospital basically tried to charge a second time for the copay and tried to justify it as more the patient owed. She was upset with the situation. Both she and her husband had to get the insurance company and the hospital on the phone in a conference call before they could get it resolved. If it happened to her, I have no doubt it has happened to many others.

One thing you will want to do is check your bill for errors, particularly if you are paying out-of-pocket. Errors do happen, and rarely are they in the patient's favor. Interestingly, insurance companies are often not at all concerned about these types of errors.

For you as a patient, whenever you can plan in advance, you want to check a hospital's reputation as well as that of its doctors. You may also want to do some comparison price shopping. Sometimes, your insurance company has already dictated your choice of places, and they will make recommendations for you. You will be limited to their choices if they are going to pay the bill. It is important, however, to be aware that shopping around is an option that can sometimes not only save you money, but can give you better care.

Companies that self-insure will do comparison shopping, and often find a better hospital that will treat at a lower price, and they will utilize those services. An interesting trend that is happening now, especially for people who pay out-of-pocket, is to go to centers in other countries that specialize in certain things. Medellin, Colombia, for example, is a hotbed of plastic surgery tourism. If you scan the Internet, you can find other countries that specialize in certain kinds of medical care for the international traveler. Do be aware, however, that your own insurance, be it Medicare, Medicaid, or a private insurer, is probably not going to pay for *any* treatment done outside this country, especially an elective procedure. Buy travel insurance or be prepared to pay for care yourself if you have an illness while traveling.

Pharmaceutical Industry

Pharmaceutical companies represent a true double-edged sword in the overall issue of medical care costs. No doubt many of the medications that we have now treat illnesses early, prevent things from worsening, and prevent many hospitalizations and deaths. It is also clear from all the legal actions that sometimes they create some bigger problems than the ones they solve.

Pharmaceutical companies have, in my viewpoint, strayed quite a distance from the honorable and ethical path they used to pursue. They charge incredible amounts for new drugs, and although they blame the cost on research, the amount they spend on marketing probably *far* exceeds what they spend on research. It is also quite clear that they contribute to the "diseasing of America" not only with all the advertising where they sell the public on having diseases, but with all the problems that can arise from some of the drugs.

We have had an explosion in the number of medications just during my tenure as a physician, and it seems to grow more each year. Despite side effects, problems with medications, and the fact the costs can be high for certain drugs, the combination of multiple new meds and multiple new surgical techniques have both done a tremendous amount to help health overall. They have also often done great harm.

As a recent example, I have a patient who had done well under my care after I got her off a number of medications and stabilized her depression. In recent months, she was getting back on more medication and having more pain. She then came in with lab work that showed worsening liver and kidney function, and she was hurting all over. She was now being scheduled to be seen by a kidney doctor, a liver specialist, and a pain specialist. One of her medications, for lowering cholesterol, could account for all her symptoms, which actually began *after* she started the medicine. A few days earlier, her family doctor had come to the same conclusion and did what I planned to do—stop that particular medicine. This is a wonderful, encapsulated example of the kinds of problems that happen with medicines every single day. It is also a clear example of why you need to track all your medications and treatments and health changes over time (see www.godrjudy.com for free forms that can help you do this).

We now have standards for blood pressure, lipids, and blood sugar which require much lower levels than the standards of forty years ago. That happened on the basis of research which was, no doubt, driven by the pharmaceutical companies so they could sell more drugs. Thus, you see many cases worse than the one above, because people are overtreated or even inappropriately treated to achieve unrealistic standards. Furthermore, recent research is suggesting that cholesterol is not the culprit in hardening of the arteries, after all. It is related to immune system issues affecting the integrity of the blood vessels' linings; it is related to having a healthy mindset.

There was a time when a great deal of medical research, pharmaceutical and otherwise, was funded by various branches of the National Institutes of Health. Now, most of the research is funded by drug companies and conducted by doctors either in their direct employ or funded by their grants, which makes the impartiality of their research questionable at best. When they fund the research of people who are also teaching about the drugs, and the companies are running huge ads in the journals that publish the articles about the drugs, it raises concern about how there can be any shred of objectivity. When these are the same doctors who teach in medical schools and the same journals that form the foundation for medical education, it displays a pattern of pharmaceutical companies having way too much influence over the direction of medical care.

Although medical journals may protest that they do a tremendous amount to weed out things (which they do) and to be unbiased (which they do), there are still problem issues, such as that those same pharmaceutical or equipment companies may be supporting that journal with advertising. Again, it becomes difficult to be truly objective.

When the price for a single dose of some drugs is almost as expensive as a hospital stay, things have gone to an unhealthy extreme. The advertising that they do puts old-time snake-oil peddling to shame with commercials cleverly crafted to make people think they just have to have a certain medication. You cannot pick up a magazine or turn on the TV or go on the Internet without getting hit with a barrage of pharmaceutical ads. I personally think the system worked much better for the *patient* when the research was more objective, billions were *not* spent on advertising to the public, the information was disseminated to doctors who then decided whether to use the medication, based on more impartial research information, and things were not so outrageously priced. Interestingly, it was the Food and Drug Administration who approved all this public advertising in 1999 over the objections of the American Medical Association and many other entities.

While I realize the current system works well for the drug companies, there has also been too much evidence that they are willing to put out medications that are dangerous and/or inadequately researched for the sole motivation of making a profit, no matter who it hurts. This is a pendulum swung too far and is adding a huge segment to the overall cost of medical care, some of which needs to be seriously pruned away. There are several books documenting these problems in much greater detail. *Inside the FDA* by Fran Hawthorne and *Bad Pharma* by Ben Goldacre are only two of many examples.

Medical Equipment Industry

The companies that manufacture medical equipment—whether it be simple home health aids like nebulizers, canes, walkers, and wheelchairs; complex items like MRI machines, positron emission tomography (PET) scanners, gamma knives, and da Vinci Surgical System robots; more personal items like artificial joints, heart valves, and prostheses; or simple devices like syringes, needles, IV tubing, hospital gowns, and bedding—produce equipment that is quite pricey. Many of the improvements in technology work well for improving patient care and bringing down the recovery time and the overall cost of things like time away from work.

However, the price of much of this equipment remains quite high. In looking at various kinds of equipment in hospitals, labs, offices, and so on, it appears to be a market that prices itself much on the high side for nearly everything, even considering the more stringent manufacturing codes. You need to realize that these companies are not working only in our best interest.

A physician colleague revealed to me that a replacement heart valve costs $5,800 in our country and a mere $500 in China. The heart valves in both countries are manufactured by the same company. (That $500 in China, though, does represent one or more months of work for some of the lower priced laborers.) I am aware from equipment pricing by myself and colleagues that electronic medical billing and record systems can cost anywhere from $3,000 to over $25,000 as a start-up cost, although cost and quality do not correlate.

If we are looking at that kind of price markup across the board, this does indeed become a major player in an industry that is managed as big business that is looking out only for its own interests. Be aware that companies work to get equipment manufactured at the cheapest price possible, but they don't do that to bring you a product at a more reasonable price, they do it to increase their profit margin, whether it is in Medicine or any other field. You need to follow the rule of "let the buyer beware" in your medical care as much as with any other kind of business you may deal with.

You, as a Consumer

The biggest problem with patients who run up medical costs is that patients fail to take adequate care of themselves, both in terms of preventing health problems and in terms of taking good care of themselves physically and emotionally when they have medical problems so they can minimize the need for additional care. At the same time that consumers are shifting to things like organically grown foods and putting in their own gardens, they still leave too much of their health care in the hands of the medical system, because they don't put effort into self-care and preventive behaviors. In addition, a patient often thinks she has insurance, is entitled to it, and plans to get everything from it she can, whether she needs it—or not. This runs up excess medical care bills with no real benefit, and sometimes with great detriment.

9

The Many Important
Issues with Medications

Antibiotics: Benefits and Life-Threatening Dangers

Basics

One basic principle I was taught in medical school was that you do *not* treat an infection—*any* infection—without *first* ordering a culture and sensitivity. This means you take a specimen, grow the organism causing the disease, and then determine what antibiotics will kill it. You also instruct your patient to take the full dose prescribed when the medicine is given, rather than stopping it once they feel better. When you culture an infection, then if the initial antibiotic that you start is not the right one, you can change it within a few days In the most dramatic illustrations of this, a patient will *not* get better—and might even get worse—if initially placed on the wrong antibiotic.

My first, and vivid, illustration of this came in my third year of medical school. A woman presented to the ER after having been bitten when she inserted her arm between two fighting cats. The ER doctor treated her with an antibiotic and sent her out. She returned *a few hours later* because her arm was already getting much redder and swelling severely. She was seen by the head of infectious disease, who did the proper, although difficult, procedure to culture a wound that was not yet forming obvious pus. The woman had an organism called *Yersinia multocida* growing in her arm. It is a common organism in cat's mouths and first cousin to the bubonic plague, an organism that killed millions of people in the 1400s and still infects a few people each year. She was then placed on the proper antibiotic as an IV. Within a few days, she was well. Without that proper treatment, she might well have been dead.

The Antibiotic Time Bomb

With the advent of antibiotics (which only really began during World War II), we have developed a serious problem that is incubating an infection time bomb that could well erupt into an epidemic of infections that will be untreatable. We have too many more organisms that have developed immunity to even multiple antibiotics. While it may sound like the theme for a Stephen King or Michael Crichton novel, it is frighteningly true. It raises the specter of an army of Typhoid Marys, carrying an infection that they do not succumb to themselves because their body is resistant to it, yet it is an infection that is resistant to antibiotics and thus spreads to a wide number of other people who do not have her resistance. (Typhoid Mary was a cook who had a salmonella [think current-day chicken products] organism causing typhoid fever. It lived in her gallbladder and allowed her to spread the disease around to many people in her city.)

We actually have examples of this floating around now. One is an infection now referred to as *methicillin-resistant staphylococcus aureus* (MRSA). It used to be called "hospital-acquired *Staphylococcus*," because—initially—most people picked it up in hospitals. Now, however, it is out and about in the community, and you might catch it from anyone who has an open, chronic wound, or even who sheds it from their nose or pubic area. You cannot tell which of these wounds are MRSA and which are something innocent, and may get infected yourself before you realize you have been exposed. Many people with these wounds are careless, even though they know they have them, especially people like drug addicts who are sharing needles and who knows what else.

Another example which has caused recent memos from CDC and occasional news stories is enteric pathogens. These are pathogens that grow in your gut or your urinary tract (and sometimes other places), and we now have strains of *E. coli*, particularly, that are being rapidly spread and are resistant to most antibiotics. *C. difficile* is another cause of diarrhea that is highly contagious and can be quite deadly. There are so many cases that are resistant to antibiotics and probiotics that they are even performing fecal transplants in extreme cases to save lives.[3] I am also seeing recent evidence of many people who are developing a pneumonia that gets extremely serious, even deadly, very quickly, and even in young, healthy adults. For others, it may only be a course of several weeks in the intensive-care unit, getting IV meds and other aggressive treatment to survive. It is distressing that these things are getting more frequent.

There are more and more people who develop these infections so severely that they can only be treated with an IV course of our newest and toughest antibiotics. Some have run out of all options. Drug companies are running out of new inventions in the antibiotic arena, and the new possibilities are at an all-time low.

---

3   See medpagetoday.com, accessed May 15, 2013.

How is this infection time bomb coming about? There are many contributing factors, most of which boil down to lack of knowledge (ignorance), taking short cuts (laziness), wanting to cut costs (cheapness), and wanting to push an array of new drugs without adequate proof of effectiveness (greed). Because it is somewhere between difficult and impossible to sort each threat out individually, I will give you some scenarios of different kinds of cases where it occurs. You can connect the dots from there and better understand the problems.

First, let's start with a problem many of you will already be familiar with. When you take an antibiotic, it is not at all unusual for you to then develop an infection you didn't count on — like the yeast infection that can you give terrible discomfort, whether it affects your mouth, your vagina, or your anus—and which requires its own treatment to clear up. This happens because when you take an antibiotic aimed at bacteria, as that bacteria is killed off, it makes it easier for other microscopic organisms, like yeast and normally helpful bacteria that normally grow in our bodies and viruses to grow more abundantly, even excessively. There are billions of bacteria we normally have in our bodies, that help our body function normally, and they can also get killed off by the same antibiotic or mutate to something problematic. In a somewhat similar way, these normal flora bacteria help defend the body from other bacteria, fungus, and probably even viruses that are around in the environment— the things that normally would not cause an infection, but now jump into that empty space and start growing wildly.

We also see this happen if we use medications that diminish our immune system function, especially in people who are on medications for things such as autoimmune diseases, or have immune system problems like HIV, or have had transplants or are on cancer treatment. These issues not only allow normal bacteria to develop resistance to treatment, but it allowed those atypical bacteria to get out of hand when we didn't have antibiotics to stop them, so we now have many organisms causing infections that were not a problem 40 years ago.

The Human Element in Infection Problems

The first element to look at here is the number of doctors who, for whatever reason, do not obtain a culture and sensitivity on the patient who has a problem before they start an antibiotic. Sometimes, it is done for lack of a handy lab facility and the sense a patient won't follow through anyway. Sometimes, they think they know what is happening, or "it's going around in the community," or they don't want to be bothered, or they want to do something quickly. Sometimes, it is because they make money from giving injections. All too often, however, it is because they cave in to the expectations—and even demands and threats (like listening to a patient who is threatening to report the doctor to the licensing board, or to sue them) of the patient who thinks she knows what she needs for some reason, such as: "I've had this before, and I know what works," or "I've been around people who had this problem, and it worked for them," and so on.

I cannot make those doctors meet what I was taught as the "proper standard," although Medicare is now pushing much harder to make that happen. I can educate you so that you know what is really going on and don't become your own worst enemy in this effort to overcome disease. The first thing you need to know is to quit demanding antibiotics for things because you *think* you know the cause and the solution, or because some TV commercial told you it was the solution to your problem.

First, not all things that seem to be infections actually are, despite the fact they cause you pain and discomfort. Certain issues, like sore throat, bladder infection, cough, wound, diarrhea, vaginal drainage or other type of complaint, are *not only* not caused by the same bacteria, but they may not be caused by a bacteria at all. Second, even if it actually is an infection, it could be a virus, a fungus, worms, a parasite, or some other infectious entity that may require a treatment that is different from standard antibiotics. In these cases, antibiotics will not only have no positive effect, but they could have a negative effect.

If an infection in a given area recurs, that suggests that other issues are going on. I listened to one female patient angrily tell me that, at her age, she knew what was going on in her body and should be able to just get what she wants for treatment from the doctor. In fact, she felt she should be able to treat herself without the aid of a doctor. She knew when she had a certain kind of infection coming back, what it was, and what would work for it.

While that is a common mindset, there are many flaws with it. First, your body does change with age, so the symptoms you have when you are younger may represent something totally different when you are older. Second, if you are having repeated episodes with the same infection—whether close together or not-so-close together—something is wrong. The right antibiotic should wipe it out, and it should not return! That becomes all the more reason to go in and have things checked more carefully, not to get lax and say "It's just that same old UTI again," or something similar.

What else could it be? It could just be coincidence that your first episode responded to the antibiotic, because it might not even have been an infection. There is a standing joke in medicine that: "I can give you an antibiotic that will make that go away in one week, or you can leave it alone and it will go away in seven days." It could be that you have something like diabetes that makes you more vulnerable to infection and needs additional treatment. It could be that you are developing a resistant strain of bacteria or that you are now developing a different kind of infection.

If everything that had four hooves and galloped was a horse, identifying them would be easy. Unfortunately, not everything in medicine is that simple.

Examples of Common Problems

UTI

Let's take a simple example of how this problem of worsening infections by use of antibiotics occurs by looking at the problem of UTIs. Patient X gets a UTI, and either calls her doctor or goes in to be seen, and states that she has a UTI and gets placed an antibiotic that *usually* works. This is done without any culture or sensitivity being done. Too often, the patient calls back, *demanding* the doctor prescribe a certain antibiotic and gets nasty when it is refused for good reason. Sure, this is fast, easy, saves the cost of the tests, and *if* it is the *usual* infection, it will *probably* clear up. However, if you don't take the full dose of medicine, or if you have already been treating that same problem with the same antibiotic and now it is coming back, the chances are increasing that you had previously killed off those bacteria vulnerable to that antibiotic. Now, because of selection and mutation, the bacteria multiplying in your system are the ones that weren't killed off. They were a little bit different; they are tougher and are becoming "resistant" to the antibiotic.

Bacteria grow and multiply quickly. They can thus change or mutate just as quickly as within the course of a day. Not only is that happening, but other bacterial species now find it easier to move in if they are not vulnerable to that antibiotic.

I see people in our psychiatric hospital, many of them coming from nursing homes, where this pattern has happened. I just saw two different cases recently infected with bacteria I had never even heard of before, bacteria that were taking over and causing the infection. It was caused by repeatedly giving antibiotics that were no longer working.

Patients come to our hospital because their mental function changes. In this case, it is because of the infection. When these patients get an adequate culture and sensitivity, we find infections that now require adequate amounts of much stronger antibiotics that must be given either intramuscular injection (IM) or an IV to kill the infection. Once bacteria develop resistance to those few antibiotics, if the infection hasn't been adequately killed off, patients are likely to die. In addition, the bacteria can get spread into the environment through the many ways that bacteria spread themselves around, and then other people are at risk as well to catch a difficult-to-treat infection.

Strep Throat

Strep throat is less of a problem since the strep test was developed, so that people don't get unnecessary treatment. Patients are warned to take the full ten-to-fourteen day course of antibiotics when it is needed. Those people who quit taking it early because they are feeling better and assume they are well, risk the possibility their own infection will return with a form that is more difficult to treat. In the case of strep throat, inadequate treatment also makes the patient more susceptible to infection of kidneys and/or heart valves, and it can turn that sore throat into a serious or even lethal disease. Shortened treatment kills the weaker bacteria and allows the tougher ones to prosper even better.

Other types of sore throats and ear problems often get treated rather quickly with antibiotics by some doctors, despite the fact they may not be from a bacterial infection at all and will not be helped by an antibiotic. Sometimes, this happens because a patient expects an antibiotic, or even demands one be given. When problems like ear or throat pain keep coming back repeatedly, it is well past time to be looking for that other something that is causing the problems, rather than continuing to treat in the same old way that isn't working. If you are lucky, the infection is a virus that can clear with the tincture of time. Some of those viruses can be treated, but with a different group of medications. Sometimes, it is a fungus that needs yet another totally different treatment. Sometimes, it isn't infectious at all. For example, allergies can cause a wide array of symptoms, and they won't respond to any of the treatments for infectious diseases.

Other Infections

Pneumonia, diarrhea, abdominal infections, skin wounds, post-operative infections, abscesses, and many more types of infections can contribute to the resistant bacteria problem. The news media frequently raises a level of panic about the latest exotic strain of influenza, or avian flu, or hantavirus, or Legionnaires' disease causing a potential worldwide epidemic. Despite the fact that we have *nearly* eradicated smallpox, polio, typhoid fever, and bubonic plague, which were all issues of the past, the real possibility exists that we will run out of effective antibiotics for some of the other microorganisms that used to be routine and easily treatable. It is now things like *E coli*, *C. difficile*, MRSA, and other previously common and easily treated infections that may well erupt into a worldwide "plague."

What Can You Do to Help Yourself?

Your role for minimizing risks for yourself and your loved ones is to use antibiotics as little as possible and *always* take them for as long as is prescribed. Be sure you get a culture and sensitivity done *before* you start the antibiotic. That way, if things do not clear up, you can quickly get on a different medication, if indicated. You need to raise questions about antibiotic treatment, if it is going on for several weeks instead of several days. Do not assume that every time you have some infection you need to go on an antibiotic. Do not insist on getting it when you are told you don't need it. Some people demand an antibiotic even after a doctor has patiently explained to them why jumping in and taking one when it isn't truly needed can cause more harm than good.

In my view as a physician, patients would be much better off demanding that their   infection be cultured before starting an antibiotic, rather than calling and demanding they be placed on a particular antibiotic. Generally going into a doctor's office with a good history and a sense of cooperative working together should be the optimum goal here.

Dangers of Taking Too Many Different Medicines

My medical school was conservative and educated us to understand that by the time you take three or more medications *of any sort* you have a 100 percent chance of a side effect or an interaction. I find this a useful rule of thumb. While it is healthier and more economical for you, it is certainly not what the pharmaceutical companies want. They want to sell you another pill, and the more expensive it is, the happier they are. And when you are taking a lot of different pills, they are ecstatically rolling in their money. Watching my colleagues, it would appear many of them have been taught the pharmaceutical industry approach to medications. The insurance companies want to fix everything possible with a pill when possible because that is cheaper than tests, surgery, etc. However, they do want you to use the cheapest meds possible.

When I began my psychiatry residency, I had many patients admitted who were on long lists of medications and had been for years. For many of them, I stopped any medication that wasn't life threatening, and often that was enough by itself to fix their psychiatric problems. It also often led to needing fewer of the other medications. That has been a practice I have followed throughout my career and still have many patients who become quite grateful when they become better with fewer medications.

However, do not undertake stopping your medications on your own. Always do it under the supervision of a physician, because you are not educated to know which things could be life threatening and which aren't. I frequently see patients making return trips to the hospital, because they decided they no longer needed any of their medications, no matter what they were for, and they wound up back in the hospital.

This is just as true for the diabetic patient and the patient with high blood pressure as it is for anyone on a psychiatric medication.

Medication Reactions

You should keep in mind that almost any kind of reaction can happen with any given food, herb, medication, beverage, etc.—ranging from good ones to bad ones. There is always a risk of those really bad allergic reactions, like difficulty breathing, or a whole body rash, or passing out, or mental changes—for these you want to go directly to the emergency room. Fortunately, those rarely happen, just like the whole body life-threatening reaction to bee stings rarely happens. Most reactions that occur are much milder, causing any of a wide array of uncomfortable or unpleasant problems. When they do occur, the proof that a new medicine is involved in the reaction you are having is that the problem goes away when you stop the medicine, and returns when you start it again. Many reactions consist primarily of rash and itching. Those reactions are easily treated by stopping the medication and taking something simple like Benadryl (unless you are allergic to *that*).

As strange as it may seem, when dealing with the tremendous variation in people's makeup, some people are allergic to Benadryl, which is to treat allergies. They can also be allergic, or have other bizarre reactions, to steroids, which are also normally used to treat allergic issues. The most bizarre reaction to steroids is to actually become psychotic. They may have hallucinations, personality changes, get confused and disoriented, and have other reactions most people, including the doctors, don't want happening. Even rice, which is a bland food that doesn't usually cause problems, *can* have adverse and allergic effects in some people.

When a problem happens that might be medication-related, the first step is to look at *new* medications that can cause their own problems and/or cause interactions with other drugs. It is also important to look at other changes that could cause problems like changes in foods, soaps, and makeup, or exposure to other chemicals, such as insecticides. It always amazes me that people on psychiatric medications are often quick to finger *those* drugs as the source of their problems, even though they have done well on them for years, rather than looking at newer meds and med changes.

While adverse reactions do occur from some medications just related to taking that medicine over a long period of time, either because of some effect that compounds over time or because your body chemistry changes as you age, allergic reactions to medications you have taken for a long time do not happen often. However, they *do* happen, and they should not be overlooked as a possibility. Our bodies change over time, and not only are the dosages of medicine different at different points in our lives and with different body sizes, but as we age our chemistry changes so that a medication that used to work well can now cause bad effects and need to be replaced with something else.

One example of changing effects as we age is with a group of medications referred to as "anticholinergic compounds." These are medications that tend to cause issues with increased pulse and blood pressure in the course of doing their job. This becomes a problem for people who, as they age, are developing problems like high blood pressure, heart disease, strokes, weight gain, dry mouth, constipation, and so on. They can also cause sedation and dizziness, which can increase risk for falls and other accidents. They includes a wide array of medications that can include OTC sleeping meds that contain Benadryl, some of our old tricyclic antidepressants, some stomach medications, bladder control medications, muscle relaxers, and an array of other medications. Some medications for Alzheimer's disease also fall in this category and can sometimes make the patient's behavior or dementia worse because of the side effects. Not only can the individual medication cause a problem, but if you wind up on several meds with these same effects all at the same time (like what happens when different doctors are treating for different things and aren't aware of everything you are taking), you can develop serious problems.

More troubling are the problems that may not show up until a medicine has been out for months or even years, such as Vioxx, which was a great pain medication—except for the increased rate of heart attacks with it. There was also the fen-phen combination for diet that caused pulmonary hypertension, so you might lose weight, but you might also lose lung and vascular function. You can watch TV, read the news, and see the medications that have been found to be so bad they are pulled off the market. Sometimes, the pharmaceutical company knew the risks were there and chose to market it anyway. Often, they were also studied for too brief a time before approval to see the longer term benefits and problems. A six-week study is hardly adequate for a medication you may need to be on for years.

Another issue that comes to mind is aspirin, which is a good medicine. When given to children with a viral infection, it can cause a complication called Reye's syndrome which can be quite serious. That is why aspirin is no longer used with babies and small children. When taken in excessive amounts, it can kill you or your kidneys, especially when it was combined with phenacetin in the old aspirin-phenacetin-caffeine analgesic compound.

You are probably aware of all the law firms advertising and advising you to sue if you have serious side effects or complications from medications, medical devices, medical procedures, etc. They do not, of course, limit themselves to the medical field. While *some* of these lawyers are little more than vultures and are strongly disliked even by their colleagues, many of them have integrity and serve a good purpose. (Yes, vultures do have benefit.) Without this cadre of lawyers, we would have many more damaging medications, products, and procedures released on the market, and many more doctors would be continuing to practice, despite being impaired or incompetent, and many more things would happen in medicine and elsewhere that shouldn't.

Medicine is much like most other fields where the good, the bad, and the ugly all exist and compete for your attention and your money.

Part of the purpose of this book is to help you be an informed, involved, watchful patient so that you never wind up in a situation so desperate that you must resort to utilizing a lawyer to gain payment for a wrong done to you. Sadly, you must be watchful in selecting a lawyer in that kind of situation also, because just as with every other field, there are the good, the bad, and the even worse than ugly.

Do Not Use TV for Your Medication Education

The advertising of medications has gotten to the level of snake-oil peddling and has been that way basically since pharmaceutical companies were first allowed to advertise in the public media in 1999. The advertising is cleverly crafted to list symptoms that are vague enough to apply to almost anybody and to any disease, so that you soon begin thinking that you have disease X and, therefore, you must need drug Y. Basically, they sell you a disease, so you will buy their medicine. Advertisers know that people are vulnerable to an easy sale when it comes to issues of health.

Sex certainly sells things even more readily, and it will often be tucked into medication advertising whenever possible, just like ads for everything else. It is overdone when it comes to selling meds to enhance sexual function. The quoted data is often shaky and biased at best whether it is what they present to you as the public, or what they present to physicians to induce us to prescribe their product. While some companies and products are good, effective, and ethical, others are not, and you must always be on your guard. Doctors also have to be on guard and watchful about what is being presented by the drug reps and in the brochures, as there is often a sleight of hand in the drug rep's presentation. They will also try to get doctors to make comments about their usage of a drug so they can go around making claims about how other doctors are using and liking their drug. I often explain to drug reps that I don't care what their clinical trials show or what they are telling me about how the drug works chemically (because I know how deceptive the information can be). I only care what happens when my patient takes it, whether good or bad, and that will determine further use, or non-use of their product.

Know What Medications You Are Allergic To

To be an informed patient, you need to know what medications you are allergic to, including OTC meds. It is also important to recognize that sometimes it is other things in a medication that have an adverse effect, such as certain food dyes, binders, and fillers that may go into them. A useful drug can sometimes be obtained free of these other elements. Learn the difference between a true allergy, a side effect, and just not liking something about the medication. Allergic reaction does *not* mean that you didn't like the taste of it or got some side effect that might be expected from a medication, like sleepiness or dry mouth.

A *true* allergic reaction occurs when you get a rash, difficulty breathing, nausea/vomiting, rapid mental changes, or some of the more severe consequences that can cause significant harm to you. You always need to report these to your doctor, and then recheck to make sure you don't accidentally still get prescribed something you shouldn't be getting. I see patients frequently complain that they are allergic to a medication when that is clearly not what the problem is. That often then eliminates a whole spectrum of medicines from use when they don't need to be. I have also had patients claim allergy to a medication just because they don't want to take it, which can be unwise, or as a way to try to corner the doctor into giving them a drug of choice (such as a narcotic), which might not be in the patient's best interest.

Side effects are a different set of reactions that can be expected to occur in a percentage of the patients taking a given medication. They can also be important and may, at times, be severe enough to warrant listing the medicine as something you don't want to take the again. Even some side effects *can* be life-threatening, but that isn't nearly as frequent as with the allergic reactions. Certainly, listing any serious side effect is important.

Things you don't *like* about a medication, such as that it tastes funny, the pill is too big, or it make you feel sleepy, and a long list of other complaints, are sometimes things that can be worked around and sometimes things you just need to live with, but they should never be reported as an allergy.

As more pharmacies and doctors go to electronic prescribing, allergic reactions, drug interactions, and age-related concerns will be checked automatically once your information has gone into your computer record. However, it is still important for you to be actively aware of your allergies. Don't hesitate to remind your doctor about them when prescriptions are being written. Also, don't hesitate to bring it up with the pharmacist if you are concerned.

Getting Off Medications

Some medications, like antibiotics, are normally prescribed to only be taken for a few days and then stopped. *However,* when they are prescribed for a certain number of days, they *need* to be taken for that number of days even if you feel better, especially medications that are taken for infections. Failure to complete the full cycle of medication may leave behind some of the stronger bacteria. They can then create a strain that is stronger and cannot be killed with that same antibiotic and are also harder to kill with the next antibiotic.

Some medications are prescribed to be taken PRN, which means "only as you need them." This includes things like headache pills, sleeping pills, or some pain pills, and you have total control of those unless you start taking them excessively. Even OTC medications, such as aspirin and some vitamins, can be a problem if you take too much of them. Of course, abuse of some other PRN substances—such as pain medication, alcohol, street drugs, and even more benign medications — can cause a problem when taken in excess.

Stopping medications too early or when not advised can be risky, and it should be done in consultation with your prescribing physician. All too often a patient thinks that because they have taken the medication a while and are now feeling better, they are cured and don't need the medication any more. In many cases, it is only because you continue to take the medication that you continue to do well and have your problem under control. There are also those situations where, if you take your medication for a while and you also work with your doctor to change behaviors that are contributing to your problem, you may be able to get to the point you no longer need medication. For example, if you learn skills to control your anxiety, you may no longer need your anxiety medication. If you work to control your weight and exercise properly, you may be able to come off meds for diabetes, blood pressure, or lipid problems. Whether you improve enough to get off medications will be determined by you and your doctor monitoring the issues involved for your particular illness.

Other problems, like an under-functioning thyroid, will likely require medication for the rest of your life, even though the dosage may need to be adjusted from time to time; there are many illnesses that fall in this category. There are also specific types of psychiatric medications that will probably need to be taken your whole life, such as meds for schizophrenia or bipolar disorder. Failure to take these medications usually winds up causing repeated hospitalizations to get the illness back under control. Working closely with your doctor and your meds will help you to function well and stay out of the hospital—well worth the effort unless you just like to stay in the hospital.

I have seen many patients be conscientious and learn the skills to take better care of themselves and thus be able to minimize or even eliminate the need for some medications, as well as diminish the need for emergency visits and hospitalizations, but this work should be done by having your doctor verify things are moving along well. A positive, can-do attitude on your part will go a long way toward helping you take better care of yourself and thus need less medication and less medical care.

If your doctor is unwilling to talk to you or work with you on the concept of decreasing medication and can't give you a good reason why, it may be a good idea to get a second opinion—just to be sure.

10

Do Your Part in Managing Your Health—and Your Disease

There is a rule of thumb in medicine that 10 percent of the patients have 90 percent of the diseases. While this may be a bit of an overstatement, it is still clear that many people have a generally good health and lifestyle. Another cadre seem to go from one illness to the next to the next and seem to stay ill most of their lives. (They are often also jumping from one emotional catastrophe to the next.) You can look at all kinds of factors that play into this, including economic status, education, where you live, what health care you have available, and so on. The bottom line to my observing eye is that those who *choose* to take reasonable care of themselves physically and mentally, no matter what the other variables are, tend to be the ones who have significantly less illness than those who do not look out for their physical and mental health. These are the people who, when they do have an illness, go to the doctor, get care, and do their part in making sure they follow the treatment plan and monitor their disease, so it is controlled. They live longer and have fewer complications of their illness.

Even for this group, their ability to do well can be compromised if they let themselves be overwhelmed with emotional issues or if they get to the point in their lives where they feel they no longer have a point or purpose in their lives. This latter issue is why, statistically, the average life span after retirement is three years. Those who have plans, goals, and purpose in their life—both during their working life and after retirement—tend to keep going long and well for *many* years after their retirement with a happy, healthy lifestyle.

Among those who don't do well are patients who have readily treatable diseases who repeatedly do not adhere to their treatments, don't take good care of themselves in other ways, and wind up back in the doctor's office or the hospital repeatedly. Too many people don't manage their diabetes at all well, despite instructions and assistance. They simply won't check their blood sugars, take their medication, exercise or avoid excess sweets. Even hospital patients often argue about treatment, and they sneak around to get things they know they should not have (like sugar for diabetics or cigarettes for pneumonia patients). They don't want to do the basic health management, wanting the doctors to cast a spell so they can do anything they want and stay healthy.

Similar issues are present for high blood pressure, some of the other cardiovascular diseases, lung disease, cancer, substance abuse (including smoking, drinking, and drugs), and mental health. One of the most difficult issues comes from people who won't give up their addictive behaviors but keep coming in for treatment of the consequences. To see anyone near death because of an illness that was totally in their control to treat or prevent and continuing to do nothing to help themselves—despite the obviously approaching consequence—is painful indeed. It also runs up the cost of medical care incredibly —not only for that patient, but for the system as a whole that has to pay for the insurance, hospitals, innovative treatments, doctors, special medical equipment, and all the other things that go into keeping each of those people alive.

The same kind of issues exist for most addictive behaviors in their own way, be they issues of food, drugs, alcohol, sex, TV, gambling, or whatever. I realize that addictions can be difficult to give up, but once you recognize your life is on the line, what keeps you from stepping up and doing what it takes? I certainly know many people who have come to that decision point and *do* make the right decision for themselves, even though it is difficult and continues to be a temptation for a long time. Some people seem addicted to not doing their fair share to help themselves. One thing I find personally most annoying are the people who have severe chronic lung disease—to the point they are in wheelchairs, on oxygen, and needing a lot of medications—who *refuse* to stop smoking! Their excuse is that it is too difficult to stop and "everybody has to die of something." Clearly, they do not want to die from the direct and indirect effects of their smoking, or they wouldn't be going to the doctor to get treatment. If giving up smoking (or any other addiction) is difficult, is dealing with your own impending death *easy?* Obviously not, or you wouldn't keep returning for help, but one of your biggest helpers has to be *you!* If it is difficult to do all those healthy things, stop and think about how difficult it is to live with pain and disability if you don't take good care of yourself.

Healthy Lifestyle

What constitutes a healthy lifestyle? While no one answer fits everyone, in my view, you do not have to go to any kind of extreme to have a healthy lifestyle. If you are emotionally content, eating reasonably, remaining moderately physically active, are happy with your work, home life, and friends, take risks to do new things but not to the point of always putting your life in peril and have a sense of goals and purpose for your life, you probably have a fairly healthy life style. While I don't advocate a style that is so middle of the road that you feel in a rut, I also don't advocate ongoing extremes of excess exercise or no physical activity, eating 200 calories a day versus eating everything in sight, or keeping yourself in a sterile environment versus exposing yourself to every noxious infectious agent you can think of. The bottom line is that if you eat to the point of marked obesity, you abuse your body by not using it and further abuse it with harmful chemicals, and the only stimulus to your brain is a soap opera on TV, you don't have a healthy lifestyle and most likely will not be healthy. Moderation goes a long way in helping you do well, but that moderation should also be punctuated with times of pushing yourself really hard and times of letting yourself be totally laid back.

Diet

Diets should *not* go to extremes if they are going to be a part of a healthy lifestyle. One reason there are so many diet programs, diet pills, and diet treatments out there is that none of them work that well for those who are trying to lose weight. They do, however, work extremely well to make money for the creator of the latest diet gimmick, exercise routine, equipment, magic formula, etc. If there were one great diet that really worked for everybody, in theory, everyone who needed to lose weight would use it and regain a healthy weight range.

I have lived long enough to see many fads come and go around the whole issue of weight management. They come and go like the seasons, and so does the weight—except that it tends to slowly, steadily still go *upward.*

Surgical procedures aren't really much better for most people. Some people will do well, and for some people they can have many complications, including death. Many surgical candidates will not lose nearly as much as they expect, and some people will wind up finding ways to totally sabotage their surgeries—even gastric bypass—and load in enough calories to stay obese. After all, beverages are not really a problem for that constricted stomach and are quickly absorbed, and some of them are high calorie. Ice cream, sweet drinks, candies, and food of that nature can also throw in many calories in a hurry. Forcing yourself to diet (and it is a horribly strict diet) by having radical surgery, rather than *disciplining* yourself to eat reasonably, just isn't a workable solution. In addition, there are many significant risks from the surgery, especially bypass surgery, both short term and long term. While the risks of surgery versus the risk of the extra weight have to both be considered, when there is a much simpler and safer way to get weight off, why risk surgery? Is it so difficult to develop some willpower and self-discipline that you would put your life at risk instead?

So what do I recommend to my patients when they want to lose weight? First, if they are fairly significantly overweight, I want them to keep a food diary to see what they are eating, when, how much, and what is going on with them emotionally when they are eating so much. It helps you get a picture of some of the things you may need to work on. Then, you can target the specific issues. If, for instance, you like to sit down and eat ice cream with your favorite TV show at night, but you can't stop without eating the entire half-gallon of ice cream—just don't bring the ice cream in the house. When you are tempted to go and get some to satisfy that craving, get yourself busy with something to take your mind off it, just like people have to do with any other kind of addiction. Once you begin to see what you are doing, you can begin to set up the strategies. If you aren't willing to do that, you have to look at why you are deliberately compromising your own health and what that is about.

Second, I recommend the standard guideline that you aim for the reasonable target of losing no more than one to two pounds a week. For various reasons, more rapid weight loss than that tends to backfire on you and ultimately interfere with weight loss and even promote weight gain. You didn't put your weight on in two weeks, so don't expect to get it off in two weeks. Also, don't expect the weight to come off in a straight line, downhill course. It will be a zigzag, up-and-down course if you are doing it right.

Third, look at the kinds of foods you like to eat and decrease the amount of them you eat. Even a 10 percent reduction in how much you eat on a daily basis will help, and you can do that. If you decrease your sweets and fatty foods, do not cut them out completely. It will help you lose weight but not leave you feeling so deprived that you give up.

My neighbor lost a great deal of weight in a way that was easy for him. He just quit eating all bread and bread-related products. It has become a lifestyle change for him for most meals, and a lifestyle change is part of what has to happen. For those of us who don't eat much bread, you have to seek other options. I, for example, love red meat and have no intention of taking it out of my diet. However, I will grill it, broil it, or bake it, rather than fry it or smother it with high-calorie sauces. But, then, I do the same thing with fish and white meat, because it lets me reduce calories while still eating something I enjoy.

Fourth, eat more things that are home cooked. Avoiding fast food, restaurant, or even pre-prepared foods from the grocery store will probably automatically decrease your calories. Those places all add salt, sugar, and fat to enhance flavor, and even if you are going with their healthy choice options, you have to be watchful. Read the labels on boxes and cans, and you will see how much sugar you can avoid by making different choices. Get a book that lists the ingredients and calories for various kinds of foods. You will be stunned at how many calories *can* be loaded into a four-ounce serving of almost anything. One of my patients shared an unusual guideline that works for her. If something has a short list of ingredients on the label, it is probably okay to eat it. If the list of ingredients is long, avoid it.

Fifth, reduce your sugar intake down to 50–100 grams a day (one Coke has 50 grams). Recognize that any name ending in "-ose," such as glucose or lactose, is a sugar, and so are things like corn syrup, high fructose corn syrup, maltodextrin, and many others. Artificial sweeteners unfortunately often add a list of problems of their own and should also be avoided. Look mostly for small amounts of natural sugars such as fruits, and use flavoring agents other than sweeteners for your beverages.

If your time is limited for food preparation, consider finding at least some things you can make in fairly large batches, freeze as individual servings, and heat up later. Basically, you are then making your own TV dinners.

In summary, cut back on fats, sugars, breads, and high-calorie beverages, and modify how you cook things. Don't try to cut those things out totally, or you will never stick to your diet. Cut back on your serving size, leave a few bites on your plate, and don't try to lose more than a pound or two a week. Don't expect things to take a steady downhill course. Your weight will fluctuate, whether the overall course is up or down the hill. Supplementing your "diet" with a good multivitamin is a good idea. You should also look for foods that are locally grown and ripened, because they maintain more nutritional value than something that is picked early, shipped far away, and then ripened artificially. The flavor will also be more satisfying.

Exercise

Exercise is a problem for many people. This is unfortunate, because generally once you do exercise you feel better, unless you start out by pushing yourself too hard and then give up. *Using* your body is really important if you are going to keep it functioning. The more you use it, generally, the better it is going to work, and the longer it is going to last. Generally, physical *inactivity* is going to *increase* a number of physical problems that would be prevented by normal usage. Not only is exercise important for our body, but it also increases the blood flow to our brain so it works better, and it helps generate chemicals that help elevate our mood so our mood is better. Our bodies were designed to be up, active, hunting and gathering food, not sitting in front of the TV with a remote control, having someone bring food and beverages to us. By the same token, we do not have to be up using heavy-duty fitness equipment or running marathons to keep in *adequate condition*.

Even many children now spend more time in that physically inactive state rather than outside playing and exercising their muscles. With the changes in foods as mentioned above, plus the decrease in exercise, it is not surprising that we now have kids who are seriously overweight even in elementary school and developing diabetes at an early age as well. Although we don't need to return to our hunter/gatherer roots, we must maintain physical activity—we must use it or lose it, and that is important throughout the lifespan.

It is fun to sit around some of the time, and it can be difficult to motivate yourself, but you need to find those ways that help you do that. It is really important if your body is going to function properly. I feel better when I exercise, and my overall energy is better, but it is tough to discipline myself to carve out time *just* to exercise—as in using my Total Gym, exercising to a video, or going to a gym. However, I do get a good level of physical activity by doing the things that I enjoy, like working in my greenhouse, which involves walking, carrying, bending, stooping, lifting, and twisting. Without even realizing it, I can get a fairly good workout and don't really work up a sweat doing it, unless it is a really hot day. There are many things that you can do that are fun and not overly strenuous, so you can do any degree of workout that you want that is enjoyable to you. Few people stick with an exercise regimen that is just really unpleasant for them, so you need to find things that are enjoyable.

I hear constantly from people all the reasons they can't exercise. Your greatest limitation is the use of the word "can't" in place of "I *can* find a way." Many exercise excuses are related being overweight or some physical illness. Unless you are paralyzed from the neck down, there are plenty of things you can do that will not stress your bad knees, your bad back, or whatever else you feel is limiting you. Swimming, water aerobics, working with hand weights while sitting in your chair watching TV, peddling a stationary bicycle—all these will give you exercise and fun. If you make up your mind to do exercise, there are other things you can come up with as a way to do exercise, instead of ways to avoid it. You don't have to do prolonged strenuous exercise—and, in fact, studies are now starting to show that just doing easier things such as the ones I do in the greenhouse, will go a long way toward maintaining fitness and help you keep weight off and feel better physically and mentally. Can it cause you some physical pain? Yes. That is a part of developing and strengthening muscle. However, as you keep doing it over a period of time the pain decreases and the function and strength increases and your body and mind function better.

Avoid Substance Abuse

There are many types of substances, both legal and illegal, that we can use that are readily available to us and can cause us great harm: some with short-term use, some with long-term use, and some with both. Ironically, some of these same substances can be beneficial when used in appropriate amounts and for limited duration, but because they are endorsed socially, considered a rite of passage, or a way to help us escape our problems, it can be tempting to turn to chemicals to modify our feelings or even to escape reality. For some people, there is a fair amount of physical or emotional vulnerability, and they can quickly get addicted to substances after only a few uses. For them, it is probably more difficult to change, but it *can* be done and *must* be done if you are not going to *slowly kill yourself* by abusing these substances.

As with issues of diet and exercise, managing this problem means *you* must decide to take better care of yourself and then decide to *do* what it takes and to follow through with it. Based on what I have observed clinically and also with computerized EEGs over the course of my career, I almost never see a pure chemical dependency. There is almost always either some significant underlying emotional issue compounded by an inability to really discuss feelings about those core issues, or there is a major psychiatric disorder, such as schizophrenia. Based on the EEG data I collected, there appears to be some decreased brain function in a particular area of the brain that showed up repeatedly in alcoholics and would correlate exactly with impaired verbal expression of emotions. Psychotherapy does help some of these people, but there is clearly also more that we need to look into here to research the cause and develop better treatment.

It can be quite amazing to watch the rapid negative emotional spiral that occurs in someone who has been clean for a while and then relapses. Their emotions and feelings reach back to some former bad emotional spot, and that is magnified many fold by the physiological effects of the chemicals that they abuse, driving them to want all the more to anesthetize themselves with their chemical of choice. Thus even a small amount of these drugs can poison their mind, making total abstinence critical for having a happy, fulfilling lifestyle.

The things that generally represent the greatest health threats to the greatest number of people in terms of drug abuse are: opiate pain medications, alcohol, cigarettes, cocaine, methamphetamine, Xanax, and some of the hallucinogens like PCP and Ecstasy. Certainly, many more things could go on the list, but those are the current major threats. More serious than any *one* of these drugs being abused is that most of them are abused in combination, allowing more death and destruction at a much quicker pace.

Opioids

One of the greatest risks to public health right now is the abuse of opioids (such as Lortab, Norco, Oxycontin, Oxycodone, hydrocodone, heroin, codeine, and morphine), which have caused a tremendous number of deaths, mostly in our younger population, but it is also an issue for the more mature population. It is now one of the leading causes of death in this country, and much of that happens from unintentional overdoses, as well as the deliberate excess doses or shooting it up just to get high. It is a medication that has been made all too readily available for managing pain. Although it is great for short-term pain management, for long-term use it generally isn't that good at pain management. It does carry a greater and greater risk of addiction, overdose, and rebound pain, as well as cloudy thinking for many people. Unlike something like cigarettes or alcohol where the time curve is long before it kills you, opiates can get to that point within a year or two.

It is important to explain the issue of rebound pain, because it causes too many good people to wind up not only addicted, but in really severe pain. That pain is often worse than the pain they started with, and much worse than they should be dealing with, based on their injuries. Basically, after the medication has been working for a while, it will start to wear off sooner. The pain may seem a little more severe as it is wearing off. This gradually becomes a vicious situation in which you are taking higher doses of the medication, and your pain remains horrible—maybe even worse than when you started. What is really sad is the number of people who find out that they are finally pain-free, or have manageable pain, once they are *off* the opiates. It is a really difficult scenario for a lot of unsuspecting people.

While the FDA is cracking down on more of the opioid abuse now, it is a long way from the kind of limitations that should happen. I hope this at least educates you and helps you make an informed judgment. If the doctor who is supplying you with those high doses of meds won't help you get off them, find a different doctor who will. If you are addicted to opiates and taking ten, twenty, thirty, forty tablets a day and/or using them IV, you are seriously putting your life at risk. You must recognize what is happening and get help getting off them. Not only are the drugs themselves dangerous, but they may be laced or cut with other things, and IV drug users have frequently had problems with those added agents as well as the opioid, and run all those other risks that come from things like sharing needles.

Stimulants

Cocaine, crack cocaine, ice, and methamphetamine (as well as Ritalin, Adderall, Dexedrine, and their various trade names) are stimulant drugs or uppers that increase your energy and your mood. When the prescription forms are used properly, they can be a positive treatment tool. Used improperly or abused, all these drugs can raise your pulse, your blood pressure, and your risk of stroke, while greatly impairing your judgment about almost everything. (Hence, the phrase "Speed kills," when you are referring to drugs.) Generally, you get a bit more warning here than with opiates. Your teeth rot out; you start having problems with hypertension; you get strokes and cardiac distress; you may get legal citations; your family or Child Protective Services may take your children away because you aren't taking good care of them; etc.

However, if you keep doing it heavily or for long, it will definitely take a toll on your physical and mental health, and I have seen it kill too many people (primarily young people). This happens directly with things like strokes, accidents, or getting killed by another drug addict. Indirect complications come when you combine it with multiple other drugs, or when the drug was contaminated with even more harmful substances, or because the users get really careless with sex or other IV drugs and contracted other diseases that can kill them, such as AIDS or hepatitis C.

The newer legal variants of these, labeled as "bath salts" or something else benign, are often chemicals that can act like a combination of some of these other stimulants, plus some hallucinogens. We see it causing really bizarre, difficult-to-manage psychoses in some people. Sometimes, we see the extreme physical aggression and/or self-mutilation like we used to see in the early days of PCP. These are not manufactured by standard pharmaceutical companies and are in no way an approved product, but they are made by the same kinds of people who run large meth labs. They manufacture in quantity and package it to sell it in places like convenience stores. (In drug-abuser circles, word spreads quickly about where and how to get any given drug.) Initially, there was no regulation of it, but it caused so many severe problems so rapidly that most states rapidly deemed it illegal and banned it. No doubt we will see other variants that cause similar, severe problems.

Alcohol

Alcohol, of course, is a socially sanctioned chemical. You will also find plenty of evidence that in controlled amounts—like a glass of wine a day (or you can take the equivalent resveratrol capsule to get the antioxidants and skip the wine)—it can be beneficial. The problem, of course, is the devastating effects when it is not controlled. It then affects not only the drinker, but family members who live with the disruptive behaviors, employers who have an employee who may be work impaired and need treatment, and of course the ever-present risk from people who drive while drinking and cause entirely too many accidents and deaths to people other than, or in addition to, themselves. As a physician, it is frustrating to see people who are literally destroying their bodies with alcohol and keep coming back in for treatment, and yet they won't do what it takes to stop drinking despite resources like Alcoholic Anonymous, rehab centers, and legal probation programs for those who have gotten DWIs.

Tobacco

Cigarettes and other tobacco products certainly are not as dramatic in their short-term detrimental effects as any of the above drugs. They can cause problems to others from second-hand smoke, and society has done much to pass rules to limit exposure of non-smokers to the negative effects of smoking. They only rarely cause a wreck when someone is fumbling for their lighter instead of focusing on the road, and they don't cause your children to be taken away. They *are* one of the most addictive substances on the planet, and it is more difficult to get people off cigarettes than it is almost any other drug. However, for the smoker, there is at least a 60 percent chance that you will get some kind of disease from smoking if you do it very long. The first risk, of course, is just the damage to your lungs that causes chronic obstructive pulmonary disease, which over time makes it more difficult for you to breathe. After that, it makes you more likely to get pneumonia and, ultimately, it makes you breathe so poorly that you have to have oxygen and are so weak you wind up in a wheelchair. Cigarettes can also lead to cancer, heart disease, and early death—shortening your life span on average about fourteen *years*. Cigars and pipes may be slightly less of a problem, but they still have the tar and nicotine that are addictive and physically detrimental.

Hallucinogens

The much-debated marijuana can make people mellow in small amounts and make you a "zombie" in large amounts. It can indeed help with pain management, as well as glaucoma management, and it reduces anxiety for some people. However, too many people spend too much time rationalizing how benign it is, while refusing to admit to some very real problems. Of course, this is mostly to justify their habit of excessive use and abuse. It *does* alter your thought processes and your judgment, and can do permanent brain damage. It can *really* do some serious damage, particularly in young people, even when it is not laced. I have seen all too many young adults who began smoking pot in elementary school and wind up looking like an atypical schizophrenic by their teens. They have hallucinations they are no longer able to get rid of.

While pot smokers may not go out and commit crimes to support their drug habit (one of the rationalizations of pot smokers), many lives are sadly wasted and written off as a mental illness, rather than a marijuana catastrophe. Many others are wasted by the total loss of motivation in life. Marijuana also often gets laced with any number of other chemicals, probably the worst of which is formaldehyde (embalming fluid) to create what is called "wet marijuana," which can really cause severe psychosis and permanent mental problems. With more medical authorization to use marijuana (and it may serve some good medical purposes in reasonable quantities), there is also more "designer" changing of the molecules—so who knows where that will lead? In the meantime, there are some synthetic legal (only because the molecule is a little different and manufactured in a lab) THC chemicals (called "K2" and other benign names, and again sold in convenience stores) that seem to get on the market. They can be problematic, because they cause a psychosis that can't be detected by current drug tests. This often leads to a misdiagnosis and excessive treatment of the psychosis as if it were schizophrenia.

Salvia, on the other hand, is a member of the mint family, and seems to be getting popular as a hallucinogen. It is usually smoked like marijuana and can cause a psychosis that is bizarre, slow to wear off, and difficult to treat with much of anything, at this point. Some of these people are severely manic and grandiose as well and are absolutely convinced they are God, even months after they have stopped smoking the salvia.

PCP (or "angel dust") and Ecstasy seem to have come back in popularity. While they can make you feel ecstatic while you are using them, they can also cause really bizarre behaviors and hallucinations.

PCP is notorious for causing severe hallucinations that are difficult to control, severe physical agitation, and self-destructive behaviors, such as pulling off body parts. Both can cause permanent damage.

Xanax

Benzodiazepines as a group (including Valium, Ativan, Klonopin, Librium, and Xanax, among others) are good medications for controlling anxiety and helping with drug withdrawal. Properly used, they serve us well. However, they also can be misused and abused. Xanax is, by far, the most addictive of the group; it wears off quickly and leaves you craving more. There is no doubt it works to help anxiety, but there is also no doubt that it is extremely addictive, prescribed excessively, and causes problems for many people, especially when they combine it with some of the other chemicals of abuse. While it may not kill you by itself, in combination it can be deadly. It can also be difficult to get people off of it, because if it is not done properly, you can have hallucinations and, possibly, also seizures. Interestingly, these withdrawal effects don't always come immediately. Sometimes, they come days and weeks later, making it difficult to diagnose what is happening without a careful history including use of all medications. Significantly, alcohol can also give a markedly delayed withdrawal reaction in some people, especially if they have liver damage.

Drug Summary

All these addictions (often to chemicals that can be helpful in low doses) and many others are harmful because they impair your quality of life, functionally, physically, emotionally, socially, and, frequently, sexually. They run up the cost of medical care for yourself and everyone else in society enormously. These costs are not just for the addictions but for all the associated illnesses and injuries to the addict and to others around them. Saddest, of course, is that it shortens your length of life and usually doesn't do much for the quality of it, either. Like so many things in life, resolving your addiction is up to you—no one else can make the decision. No one else can be tough enough to do it for you. It is your life, and your choice, but when you have this information about how destructive these things are, it is time for you to do some serious self-examination about why you are on such a self-destructive path.

There are other options to consider like getting into serious counseling and also taking up some hobbies that will absorb that addictive need without the destructive aftermath. One reason for counseling is because the vast majority of people with addiction issues are also dealing with underlying emotional issues. Getting help with those problems makes it easier to deal with the addiction rather than using the addiction to run away from the issues that are causing your pain.

Mental Health

Too many people in this world think mental health care is just for crazy people. They don't understand that everyone's mental state is important to his own *physical* well-being and that it must be cared for just like the body must be cared for. Failure to take care of your emotional "dis-ease" can cause a wide array of pain and distress and make you much more vulnerable to acquiring physical diseases and having difficulty getting over them, as well as being more at risk for addiction issues.

Depression, particularly, is a serious emotional problem that affects 1 out of 6 people at some point in their lifetime, has a 15 percent suicide rate, and is the number 8 cause of death in the United States. When not treated it also causes high costs to society because of the medical leave time that people have to take, not just for depression, but for medical issues caused or worsened by depression. It is difficult for your body to function properly if you are an emotional train wreck.

If you are one of those "be strong" types who stuff all their feelings down like many of the characters played by John Wayne, you increase your risk to develop issues like ulcers, high blood pressure, heart attack, and similar "minor" problems. You cannot just put on a tough façade and made it all go away. Dealing with depression and other feelings does not mean you are some blubbering fool sitting on a therapist's couch. It means you learn better ways to communicate feelings, better ways to resolve problems with people, better ways to let go of those things that are eating you up inside. From there, you can move into a place of truly feeling happier and more content with your life and no longer let all "those other stupid people" mess up your life for you. If you came from a truly happy and well-adjusted family that really modeled good skills for you and didn't have problems, and if everyone around you is behaving the way you want them to so they don't cause you distress, then you probably don't have any emotional issues.

However, there is a *large* segment of the population where even though the family did the best they could to raise them, the family didn't have the skills to teach them to cope with the changes in the world now, compared to the world of fifty or one hundred years ago. We live in a world that has gone through so many changes in such a short time. All of this has had an impact on how we live, how we work, and how we play. They are changes that couldn't even be imagined by our parents or grandparents, which rather limits how they could teach us to cope with them.

Many people do things differently from the way you do them. Sometimes this can cause problems and distress for you. The positive side of that issue is that life would be really boring if we were all clones of each other. Many people get into the pattern of abusing alcohol or drugs to deal with their pain and problems, but that just adds another layer of difficult problems to cope with.

Mental health is an area where the drug companies have pushed to develop a wide array of often expensive medications. Many work no better than a sugar pill, and some have problematic side effects. Ironically, the insurance companies are willing to pay for these medications, even when used excessively, inappropriately, and in combinations that turn patients into non-functional zombies. It is also ironic that 90 percent of psychotropic medications are given by non-psychiatrists. Modern-day psychiatrists are mainly taught to give medications and not to do therapy. Part of the issue is that insurance will pay billions to keep you on drugs, but they are reluctant to pay for psychotherapy.

The good news, however, is that there is help for emotional problems; medication is *not* the whole answer. There is a big difference in the pain that comes from a physical illness and the pain that comes from years of having your personal feelings constantly under attack. There is no medicine or surgery on this planet that can turn around those thoughts and feelings related to believing your mother rejected you, or that your coworkers are making fun of you, or that you must be a bad person for bad things to be happening to you, or the long litany of thoughts we have in our head that drive us into misery.

While some medication may help temporarily, just like a cast helps with the pain of a broken arm, the healing has to come from the inside, and that happens for emotions by learning new skills from others about how to cope. Could you do it alone? You are probably about as likely to be able to do that as a brain surgeon is able to operate on his own brain. Fortunately, there are many good counselors and therapists who can really help you see where your problems are coming from and teach you more effective ways to solve your problems. There are also many wonderful books and audio programs to give you additional ideas. Think of it in terms of going to a school of personhood to learn skills you didn't learn at home, much like you would go to college to learn skills you didn't learn at home.

Learning to be mentally at ease is such an important area for our overall satisfaction in life, and it is something poorly addressed in school, home, and work environments. Good mental health is important to maintain good physical health.

Psychiatric disorders, such as schizophrenia and bipolar disorder, do require medications, usually long term, to manage symptoms and improve the quality of life. Psychotherapy still helps here to teach people ways to adjust and adapt. These patients especially are likely to be put on multiple psychiatric medications, sometimes to the point of creating a whole cadre of other problems for the patient. As with any other medical problem, the fewest number of meds in the smallest dose needed to regain control is the best way to medicate.

Summary

There is probably no health system on Earth where you cannot find both things to complain about and things to be proud of. There is no doubt that worldwide health quality has improved, and longevity has increased. Despite things moving forward, some advances bring resistance. Some advances bring new problems to solve, whether in the medical care or in the fabric of life and society as a whole. You must be careful when dealing with the problems in the medical care system not to throw the baby out with the bathwater. Rather, we should build on the strengths to start resolving the problems. Education is an important part of that process, and that is the point of this book.

When I look at health issues across the world, a few facts jump out at me. First, although we are probably the wealthiest country in the world—although there are a few small countries with a much higher per capita wealth level—and we probably have the costliest health care system in the world, our longevity ranks about thirtieth among the two hundred or so nations of the world. In addition to shorter lives, our health ranks near the bottom of the list of industrialized nations in too many areas. Second, in the past few hundred years as improvement in health and longevity have increased worldwide, it has been strongly influenced by issues that have to do with prevention, such as washing hands, clean water, sanitation, eliminating particular insects, immunization, and increased safety standards. Third, people's health is better in countries where they are more aware of good personal health care and preventive maintenance. Thus, the Japanese, who eat well, stay slim, and get more exercise, do much better than Americans and many other countries, and rank at the top in health and longevity. Fourth, people who need treatment have much better results when they are proactive, involved in their own care, and are responsible for taking their medications and/or any other treatments or lifestyle changes that are needed to help them manage their healthcare.

I have no doubt medical care costs will continue to increase for quite some time. We will continue to have many of the problems I have discussed; these problems will continue to worsen as they have over the past forty years. I also have no doubt that no matter what goes on there, if each of us does our part in better maintaining our own health, not only will that problem have less impact, but it might even help turn some of those issues around based on the free market system of supply and demand.

I hope this book proves to be a useful tool for you to get better health care by understanding more about how to navigate through the system and what and where the problems are that create frustration and increased expense not only for you, but for your physicians and for your employers, also. Things are changing rapidly. The unfortunate consequence of Obamacare is that it did not go into effect fully and immediately, thus allowing players, especially the insurance companies, to escalate their rates rapidly, to change their rules, and to decrease their reimbursements before the rules go into effect. It is not the doctors and not the federal government that is putting that kind of change into place.

In addition, I hope that learning how to navigate some of these various areas, you will learn how to get better health care at a more reasonable price and develop a good working relationship with a primary care physician. I hope you will be more attentive to taking good care of this magnificent creation known as the human body with its totally incredible human brain. We are each issued only one of them for a lifetime. If we treasure it and treat it well, it will generally serve us long and well.

Even with disease and injury, you play an important role in your survival. With the incredible things that are now available within the field of medicine, many more options are available to help you in your journey. In many ways, however, much like all other areas of life, you will get what you can afford, and most of us cannot afford a Ferrari, a Maserati, or the gullwing Mercedes. Similarly, there are many things in medicine accessible only to those who have developed the financial capability to pay for it out-of-pocket, if needed. There are two really good things about this: First, they often provide stimulus to companies to work to develop newer and better products and technologies; second, they can inspire you by example to "be all you can be," as you walk through this life. There are many things available to help you learn how to manage finances better and improve them just as this book can help you manage your health better, and I wish you well in pursuing everything that will bring you the most in your life in health, wealth, happiness, fantastic relationships, and a sense of true accomplishment for achieving those goals in an honest and socially beneficial fashion.

Bibliography and Other Resources

For those of you who wish to read further, I have placed a list of relevant books and articles I used for this book on my website. You may access it free of charge. It is at www.godrjudy.com.

At this website you will also find a variety of helpful forms available for free download, such as medical information and medical history forms, to help you take charge of your own health. There will also be other interesting and useful information on the site, so visit it frequently.

Acknowledgments

I would like to thank my son, Tom Cook, for my cover photo, and for all the support that he, his wife Sherri, my granddaughter Jane, my siblings by choice Tom and Liz Wells, and my sister Diane Bagby have been to me throughout this entire process.

Ana Lioi has been a wonderful coach who has "held my feet to the fire" to help me stay on track with the project despite my busy schedule. Thanks also to all the other folks from Peak Potentials who offered helpful information and inspiration.

My office manager and right-hand person, Crystal Jones, has been so helpful to me with her feedback, with sharing information about what she goes through with the insurance companies, and her tireless work to free me up to do my doctoring and writing.

Thanks to all the patients who helped me see the need for this book (and others that will hopefully follow) and those colleagues and friends who were so very encouraging to me about the book, especially Jennifer and Mike Harrison, Chris Skotnik, Barbara Lueking, Paula Chambers, Ana Lioi, and all the others who helped with their comments and feedback

My eternal gratitude goes to the editing staff at Amanda Rooker Editing, especially Amanda and Ben Rooker for not only their superb editing but also their patience in guiding me through the "proper" editing process.

Last, but certainly not least, many thanks to Terry Whalin, Margo Toulouse, and all the staff at Morgan James Publishing who have turned this dream into a reality.

About the Author

Dr. Judy Cook has had more than fifty years of experience in the medical field. She graduated from the University of Texas Health Science Center in San Antonio in 1973, after which she completed a pathology residency in Dallas; part of it was at Parkland, and part of it was at Baylor Hospital in Dallas. After recognizing the importance of mental health in physical illness, she changed to psychiatry and returned to San Antonio to train at the medical school and associated VA Hospital. She has been in the private practice of psychiatry since 1980, treating thousands of patients from age four and up for a wide range of problems. She has experienced the in-the-trenches issues that abound for patients, physicians, and many other components of the health care system.

She currently practices psychiatry in Sherman, Texas, and lives near there with her chocolate Labrador and a greenhouse full of orchids.

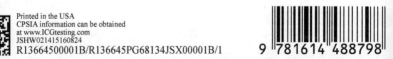

To Die, or Not to Die